ASCITES - PHYSIOPATHOLOGY, TREATMENT, COMPLICATIONS AND PROGNOSIS

Edited by **Luis Rodrigo**

Ascites - Physiopathology, Treatment, Complications and Prognosis
http://dx.doi.org/10.5772/67965
Edited by Luis Rodrigo

Contributors

Andra-Iulia Suceveanu, Despina Todescu, Filippos Manousos Goniotakis, Felix Voinea, Eugen Dumitru, Laura Mazilu, Adrian-Paul Suceveanu, Roxana Hulea, Hussien Elsiesy, Aziza Ajlan, Waleed Al-Hamoudi, Tomomi Kogiso, Kuniko Yamamoto, Mutsuki Kobayashi, Yuichi Ikarashi, Kazuhisa Kodama, Makiko Taniai, Nobuyuki Torii, Etsuko Hashimoto, Katsutoshi Tokushige, Radomir Živadinović, Aleksandra Petric, Dane Krtinic, Sonja Pop-Trajkovic, Biljana Živadinović, Emilio Fabrega, Javier Crespo, Jose Ignacio Fortea, Patricia Huelin, Alain Piché, Isabelle Matte, Bessette Paul, Asma Alnajjar, Faisal Abaalkhail, Tala Beidas, Mohamed Abdelfattah, Abdulrahman Bendahmash, Luis Rodrigo

Published by InTech

Janeza Trdine 9, 51000 Rijeka, Croatia

Publishing Process Manager Maja Bozicevic
Technical Editor SPi Global
Cover InTech Design team

First published November, 2017
Printed in Croatia
Legal deposit, Croatia: National and University Library in Zagreb

Additional hard copies can be obtained from orders@intechopen.com

Ascites - Physiopathology, Treatment, Complications and Prognosis, Edited by Luis Rodrigo
p. cm.
Print ISBN 978-953-51-3613-2
Online ISBN 978-953-51-3614-9

For EU product safety concerns:
IN TECH d.o.o., Prolaz Marije Krucifikse Kozulić 3, 51000 Rijeka, Croatia,
info@intechopen.com or visit our website at intechopen.com.

Meet the editor

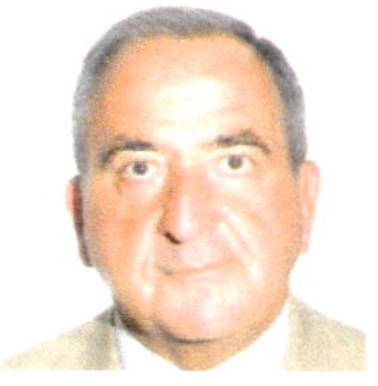

Prof. Luis Rodrigo is actually emeritus full professor of Medicine at the University of Oviedo (Spain). He has been the chief of Gastroenterology Service at the HUCA Hospital in Oviedo, for more than 40 years. He achieved his doctoral degree in 1975 and has developed a long teaching and research career during this time period. He has published a total of 565 scientific papers, of which 284 are written in English. He has directed 40 doctoral thesis, and he was the main investigator in a total of 45 clinical trials. He has contributed actively to the formation of around 100 specialists in gastroenterology. He has written around 35 chapters in books of several subjects and has been the Editor of 15 books.

Contents

Preface

Several pathogenic processes have been implicated in the development of the abdominal ascites. Portal hypertension, most usually in the context of liver cirrhosis, can explain about 75% of the cases, whereas infective, inflammatory and infiltrative etiologies can account for the rest.

The use of ascitic amylase and mycobacterial cultures/PCR when there is strong suspicion for tuberculosis and pancreatitis, respectively, helps to achieve a correct diagnosis. Ascitic cytology can be useful when cancer is suspected and has a good diagnostic yield, if it is performed correctly.

Effective treatment of the cirrhotic ascites is based on the use of a salt-free diet together with the rational use of diuretics. The most commonly used are the antagonists of aldosterone acting on the distal tubule and associated in some situations with furosemide that acts on the proximal tubular part of the kidney inhibiting the sodium reabsorption at this level. When the situation is unresponsive to diuretics, other techniques including the performance of a TIPS (Transjugular Intrahepatic Portosystemic Shunt) can be used. The correct management of ascites permits to achieve a great improvement on the quality of life and also on the survival rate.

Common complications of decompensated liver cirrhosis are esophageal varices, hepatic encephalopathy, and ascites. After the onset of complications, the prognosis notably worsens. In patients with ascites, the 5-year mortality rate is 44%. Furthermore, the presence of hyponatremia, the spontaneous bacterial peritonitis presentation, and the onset of a hepatorenal syndrome, together with an increase in the liver insufficiency degree, also greatly worsen the prognosis of the patient.

There is a general agreement about the recommendation to use cefotaxime as the first antibiotic of choice for SBP and large-volume paracentesis for the management of ascites greater than 5L in volume. For hepatorenal syndrome, cautious diuresis, volume expansion with albumin, and the use of vasoactive drugs are usually recommended. Finally, in the refractory ascites associated with advanced cirrhosis, the liver transplant performance is the best option to apply in these patients.

The great advances achieved in the last years will help to get an early and clear diagnosis of tuberculous peritonitis, due to a quick response immunological-based analysis that has permitted to get a better and early treatment for the affected patients.

In carcinomatous peritoneal ascites, there is an increasing evidence supporting an active role of the own ascites in the progression of ovarian cancer. Although much work is still needed, to fully understand the contribution of ascites to ovarian cancer aggressiveness, this tumor environment potentially provides a wealth of opportunities for translational research including biomarker discovery and novel therapeutic target identification.

I want to thank all the authors for their excellent contributions, InTechOpen editorial team and especially to Ms. Maja Bozicevic, for her continuous collaboration and kind support in the book preparation and for maintaining help all the time when needed during the editorial process.

Prof. Luis Rodrigo, MD
Emeritus Full Professor of Medicine, University of Oviedo
Oviedo, Spain

Section 1

Diagnosis and Physiopathology

Chapter 1

Introductory Chapter: Treatment of Ascites Associated with Cirrhosis and Its Complications

Luis Rodrigo

Additional information is available at the end of the chapter

http://dx.doi.org/10.5772/intechopen.70232

1. Introduction

The presence of ascites is the commonest complication in patients with cirrhosis. Approximately 60% of cirrhotics end up exhibiting it during the course of their disease. The development of ascites indicates a clear decompensation of the disease and is generally associated with a bad prognosis, with an approximately 40% of 1-year mortality [1, 2].

2. Pathophysiology

In patients with cirrhosis of the liver, a circulatory dysfunction is common, characterized by a decrease in systemic vascular resistance secondary to splanchnic arterial vasodilatation, which occurs as a consequence of portal hypertension.

In the early stages, when cirrhosis is compensated for and patients remain asymptomatic, systemic vascular resistance is low and effective blood volume and blood pressure remain normal, due to an increased cardiac output.

In more advanced phases of cirrhosis, there is progressive splanchnic vasodilatation, accompanied by a marked reduction in the effective arterial volume that can no longer be compensated for by an increase in cardiac output.

In this situation, to maintain an effective blood volume and to maintain blood pressure within normal limits, the systemic baroreceptor systems are activated, leading to the activation of the vasoconstrictor systems, including the renin-angiotensin-aldosterone system (RAAS), the sympathetic nervous system (SNS) and, in later stages, the non-osmotic hypersecretion of vasopressin.

Despite these positive effects, these vasoconstricting factors also have negative effects, especially because they facilitate the retention of sodium and water by the kidneys, influencing the appearance and maintenance of ascites, oedemas and dilutional hyponatraemia.

In the later stages of the disease, intense renal vasoconstriction occurs, leading to a significant decrease in glomerular filtration and the development of hepatorenal syndrome (HRS).

At this stage, there is also a notable drop in the cardiac output, probably arising from cirrhosis-associated cardiomyopathy, which further worsens the decrease in effective arterial volume (**Table 1**).

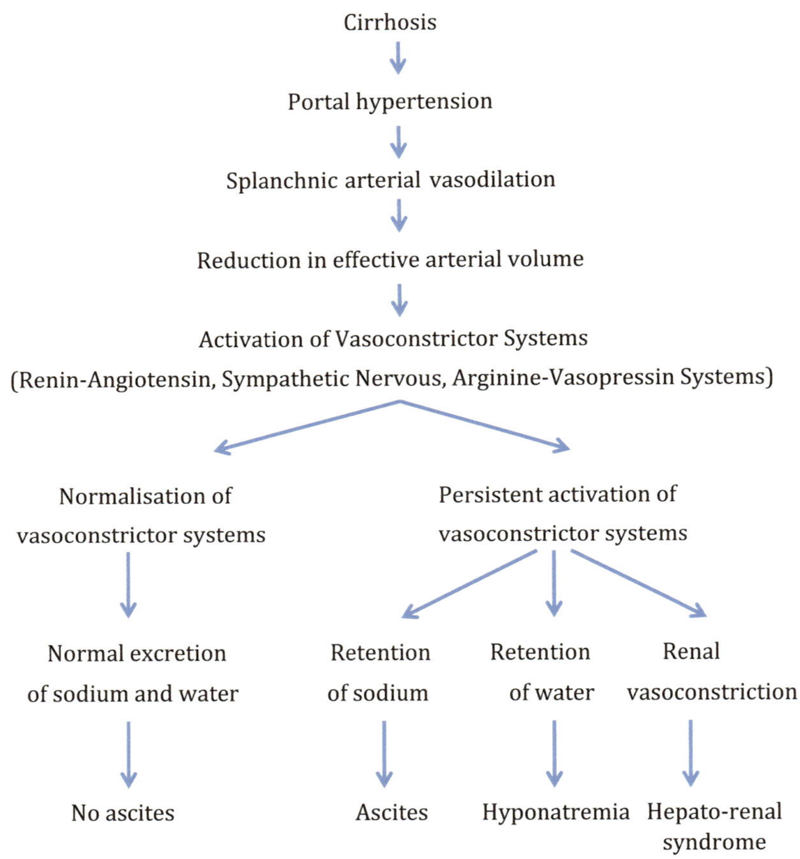

Table 1. Pathophysiology of ascites and its complications in cirrhosis.

3. Diagnosis

For every patient who attends a consultation with suspected ascites, it is essential to confirm, using exploratory paracentesis, that they have a clinical decompensation. This is irrespective of whether it is their first occasion or if they have previously had ascites. The analysis of the ascitic fluid makes it possible to rule out other causes of ascites, such as the presence of associated spontaneous bacterial peritonitis (SBP).

The diagnosis of cirrhosis is usually based on clinical, analytical and ultrasound criteria. In case of doubt, the serum albumin/ascites gradient (SAAG) should be determined. When this is greater than 1.1 g/dl, it suggests the existence of portal hypertension. Furthermore, patients with low concentrations of proteins in the ascitic fluid (<1.5 g/dl) have a worse prognosis. Likewise, the polymorphonuclear (PMN) leukocyte count is very useful for ruling out the presence of SBP; in these cases, ascitic fluid cultures must be grown in blood culture bottles.

4. Classification

The International Club of Ascites has a three-grade classification:

Grade 1: Ascites can only be detected by abdominal ultrasound, since it comprises only a small quantity or is of slight degree and is not accompanied by any clinically evident abdominal distension.

Grade 2: Ascites is usually detected by physical exploration and the patient exhibits moderate abdominal distension.

Grade 3: A voluminous ascites is present, giving rise to pronounced abdominal distension.

5. Treatment

In the absence of other, associated complications, patients with uncomplicated ascites can be treated on an outpatient basis.

5.1. Grade 1 ascites

In principle, neither dietary nor pharmacological treatments are required.

At present, there is insufficient information about its natural history and possibilities of progression.

5.2. Grade 2 ascites

This is the most common form of presentation. There is generally a moderate retention of sodium (urinary Na >20 mEq/day), without upsetting the excretion of the solute-free water and with normal glomerular filtration.

The main aim of the treatment is to achieve a negative sodium balance, to which end its oral intake must be reduced and its elimination increased by using diuretics. There is increased sodium reabsorption at the level of the distal tubule due to the presence of secondary-associated hyperaldosteronism.

Therefore, aldosterone-antagonist diuretics, such as spironolactone, are the drugs of choice and are more effective than loop diuretics.

Patients with primary ascitic decompensation should be treated with spironolactone at a dose of 50–100 mg/day and, in the event of the failure to respond, the dose should be progressively increased week by week until a maximum dose of 400 mg/day is reached.

In patients with recurrent ascites, it is recommended to combine furosemide with aldosterone antagonists. The dose of diuretics should be adjusted in order to yield a weight loss of around 500 g/day in patients who only present ascites and of up to 1 kg/day in those with associated oedemas.

As a maintenance treatment, the minimum dose of diuretics necessary to avoid the development of complications related to the treatment, such as hyponatraemia, hepatic encephalopathy or renal failure, should be recommended (**Table 2**).

5.3. Grade 3 ascites

The first-line treatment for patients with voluminous ascites consists of performing periodic evacuation paracentesis combined with administering intravenous infusions of albumin at a dose of 8 g/l of ascites removed, which is usually carried out under a regime of a short-stay admission in the day hospital.

The evacuation of a large quantity of ascitic fluid may be associated with the well-known post-paracentesis circulatory dysfunction syndrome. To prevent this, appearing infusions of albumin are administered, which reduce the incidence of complications during the following month.

After performing evacuation paracentesis with the subsequent replacement of albumin, patients must continue with a diuretic treatment of the minimum dose necessary to prevent reaccumulation of the ascites. It has been confirmed that intravenous albumin is the most effective plasma expander when more than 5 l of ascites is removed [3–5] (**Table 3**).

- Adhere to a low-sodium diet, with an average content of 80–120 mEq/day
- Initiate diuretic treatment with spironolactone (50–100 mg/day) in a single dose
- Control weight on a daily basis, maintaining a loss of approximately 500 g/day without oedema and 500–1000 g/day when there is ascites with oedema
- If there is no response, progressively increase the dose of spironolactone week by week, up to a maximum of 400 mg/day
- In non-responders, add furosemide at an initial dose of 40 mg/day, possibly increasing this up to a maximum of 160 mg/day
- Once the ascites has been controlled, administer the minimum dose of diuretics necessary to prevent the reaccumulation of ascites

Table 2. Treatment of moderate (Grade 2) ascites.

- Adhere to a low-sodium diet, with a content of less than 80 mEq/day
- Perform evacuation paracentesis in conjunction with intravenous administration of albumin at a dose of 8 g/l of ascites removed
- If the patient is not already receiving diuretic treatment, start a combined treatment of spironolactone 100 mg/day with furosemide 40 mg/day
- If the patient has previously been treated with a diuretic, restart it at a higher dose than the former one
- If there is no response, monitor the intake of sodium and increase the dose of diuretics to a maximum of spironolactone 400 mg/day and furosemide 160 mg/day
- Once the ascites has been controlled, maintain a low-sodium diet and the minimum dose of both diuretics to prevent its reaccumulation

Table 3. Treatment of severe (Grade 3) ascites.

6. Refractory ascites

This is defined as the situation in which the ascites cannot be completely eliminated or whose frequent recurrence calls for continuous medical treatment. This form accounts for approximately 10% of cases.

The development of refractory ascites is associated with a poorer short-term prognosis, the median survival being about 6 months. For this reason, all these patients, except the very elderly or those who have serious associated illnesses that contraindicate it, must be considered potential candidates for a liver transplant and should be evaluated to determine their degree of priority in the waiting list.

6.1. Periodic evacuation paracentesis

The commonest treatment indicated for patients with refractory ascites is to perform periodic evacuation paracentesis simultaneously with the administration of intravenous albumin infusions. In most cases, diuretics are not effective under these circumstances, and they must permanently cease to be used in patients who develop complications related to a diuretic treatment.

In the other patients, who maintain a level of urinary excretion of sodium greater than 30 mEq/day, the diuretic treatment may be maintained in order to delay the reaccumulation of the ascites and thereby also the need for periodic evacuation paracentesis to be performed so often [6, 7].

6.2. Portosystemic venous shunts (TIPS)

These consist of an anastomosis and an intravascular prosthesis that is introduced percutaneously by a medical expert in haemodynamic techniques. This establishes a new route of communication, at the intrahepatic level, between the portal system and the general circulation. The insertion is generally achieved by entering through the external jugular vein. This gives rise to the term for the prosthesis, the transjugular intrahepatic portosystemic shunt, and its acronym, TIPS.

After the placement, there is an increase in renal blood flow, accompanied by an increase in renal excretion of sodium, consequently giving rise to an improvement in the control of the ascites. The method is more effective than performing evacuation paracentesis for controlling ascites.

However, the placement of TIPS is associated with a higher incidence of complications, among which the most common is the occurrence of episodes of hepatic encephalopathy, as occurs in 30–50% of cases. The use of TIPS is out of the question for patients with advanced cirrhosis [8].

There are no data concerning improved survival rates, for which reason a second-line treatment is considered. It is considered to be indicated only in patients with preserved hepatic function, or when paracentesis is ineffective or has to be performed frequently (**Table 4**).

- Adhere to a low-salt diet, with a sodium content less than 80 mEq/day
- Perform evacuation paracentesis repeatedly, in conjunction with intravenous administration of albumin at a dose of 8 g/l of removed ascites
- Avoid diuretic treatment, except when no complications arise and when the patient maintains a level of renal excretion of sodium of >30 mEq/day
- TIPS can be considered as an alternative treatment for patients with good hepatic function or in whom it is difficult to evacuate the ascites by loculation
- A liver transplant will be considered if there are no contraindications and if they are on the transplant waiting list

Table 4. Treatment of refractory ascites.

7. Hyponatraemia

This is a frequent complication in patients with advanced cirrhosis and is associated with a poor prognosis. It is an important factor related to the deterioration in the quality of life of these patients.

7.1. Definition and differential diagnosis

Hyponatraemia is defined in an arbitrary manner, by the presence of a serum sodium concentration of less than 130 mEq/l. It has a mean prevalence of 22% in patients with cirrhosis and ascites. There are two varieties of hyponatraemia: hypovolaemic and hypervolaemic (or dilutional). The differential diagnosis between the two types is fundamental, since their treatment and prognosis are completely different.

7.1.1. Hypovolaemic hyponatraemia

In general, its origin is related to the loss of extracellular fluid. Patients show signs of dehydration, frequently associated with hepatic encephalopathy. Its most frequent causes are very copious diuresis, secondary to the prolonged or intense administration of diuretics, or the presence of digestive losses of fluids, in the form of vomiting or diarrhoea. Its treatment is based on controlling the cause, suspending diuretics and administering saline solutions to solve the problem.

7.1.2. Hypervolaemic hyponatraemia

This is predominant in patients with advanced cirrhosis and is characterized by the marked expansion of the extracellular volume. It arises as a direct consequence of the reduction in the capacity of the kidneys to eliminate solute-free water and is secondary to the existing circulatory dysfunction.

Its origin is probably multifactorial, although the most important factor is the presence of a non-osmotic hypersecretion of vasopressin, which acts at the level of the renal collecting tubules, causing a significant increase in the retention of free water [9–11].

7.2. Treatment of hypervolaemic or dilutional hyponatraemia

Treatment is based on increasing the excretion of retained free water, for which several options are available.

7.2.1. Fluid restriction

This remains the first-line treatment in these patients. Clinical experience indicates that such restriction prevents the progressive drop in plasma sodium levels but is not sufficient to reverse hyponatraemia.

7.2.2. Administration of saline solutions

Hypertonic saline infusion has been used, but has proved to be of little value. In addition, it is associated with two types of problem. First, their effect is of short duration and, second, sodium levels fall shortly after the treatment is discontinued. Furthermore, they increase ascites and oedema, so their administration was discontinued rapidly.

7.2.3. Albumin

Infusion of intravenous albumin is usually effective, since, being a good plasma expander, it alleviates circulatory dysfunction. However, because there have been few cases, experience of this recently established method has been very limited so far. Therefore, more studies, with a greater number of patients, are needed to demonstrate its true efficacy [12, 13].

7.2.4. Vaptanes

These are active, orally administered drugs and are selective antagonists of V2 receptors of vasopressin. They have the effect of increasing renal excretion of solute-free water. They are therefore used in different situations, such as in the treatment of patients with the syndrome of inappropriate antidiuretic hormone secretion (SIADH), in cases of heart failure and in liver cirrhosis, being effective in 45–80% of cirrhosis cases.

Its most frequent side effect is thirst. Significant increases in plasma sodium levels should be avoided, in order to prevent the appearance of neurological complications, such as central pontine myelinolysis, among others.

Tolvaptan was approved in the United States for the treatment of severe hypervolaemic hyponatraemia (Na <125 mEq/l), whereas in Europe it was only approved for the treatment of SIADH. It is mainly indicated only for cirrhotic patients who are on the waiting list for a liver transplant.

However, the US Food and Drug Administration has drawn attention to the potential risk of liver injury from tolvaptan and recommends this drug not be used in patients with liver disease [14, 15].

8. Spontaneous bacterial peritonitis

This is the most frequent and characteristic bacterial infection of patients with liver cirrhosis and associated ascites.

It is defined as the infection of ascitic fluid in the absence of an intra-abdominal focus. The most frequently associated bacteria are the enterobacteriaceae (*Escherichia coli, Klebsiella pneumoniae*, etc.) and non-enterococcal streptococci (*Streptococcus pneumoniae, S. viridans*, etc.).

In its initial stages, the patient may be asymptomatic, but characteristic symptoms, such as abdominal pain, fever, nausea, vomiting and diarrhoea, soon appear. Patients may also suffer from paralytic ileus, hepatic encephalopathy, digestive haemorrhage or renal failure.

To confirm its diagnosis, it is necessary to perform diagnostic paracentesis and undertake a cell count of the ascitic fluid.

The finding of more than 250 polymorphonuclear leukocytes/cm^3 of ascitic fluid is considered diagnostic of SBP, irrespective of the results obtained from bacterial cultures.

Once the diagnosis has been made, an antibiotic treatment should be instituted as soon as possible. Third-generation cephalosporins continue to be the empirical treatment of choice for community-acquired SBPs. In nosocomial episodes and potentially in those related to the health system, antibiotic coverage should be broader and adapted to the local pattern of resistance. The duration of the treatment is adjusted with respect to the results obtained from the paracentesis control diagnostics, continuing for up to 24–48 h after confirmation of the resolution of the infection (<250 PMN/cm^3).

It should also be remembered that patients presenting with renal and/or hepatic dysfunction at the time of diagnosis should receive intravenous albumin in order to prevent the development of renal failure and to improve short-term survival [16–18].

8.1. Primary SBP prophylaxis

Patients with a low protein concentration in the ascitic fluid (>10–15 g/dl) have a higher risk of developing a first episode of SBP, in comparison with those in whom the protein concentration remains high. In the absence of additional risk factors, the probability of developing it during the course of 1 year is less than 20%.

Evidence of advanced hepatic impairment (Child-Pugh >9 points), with bilirubin >3 mg/dl, or circulatory dysfunction (creatinine >1.2 mg/dl or a plasma sodium level of <130 mEq/l) in patients with low levels of proteins in the ascites increases the risk of developing an SBP by up to 60%.

Administration of norfloxacin at a dose of 400 mg/day in these patients reduces the probability of infection to 7%, prevents the development of hepatorenal syndrome and improves short-term survival. For this reason, it is appropriate for this subgroup of patients to make long-term use of norfloxacin, especially if they are on the waiting list for a liver transplant [19].

9. Hepatorenal syndrome

Hepatorenal syndrome is a frequent cause of renal failure in patients with advanced liver cirrhosis and is associated with poor short-term prognosis. It is a functional renal failure that develops as a consequence of intense renal vasoconstriction.

9.1. Diagnosis

There are two types of HRS: 1 and 2.

Type 1 HRS presents as rapidly progressing acute renal failure, with blood creatinine values increasing sharply to a level greater than 2.5 mg/dl. It is associated with very poor short-term prognosis, with a median survival without treatment of only 2 weeks.

Type 2 HRS is characterized by more moderate and stable renal failure, with plasma creatinine values generally ranging from 1.5 to 2.5 mg/dl. It typically occurs in patients with refractory ascites; their median survival is 6 months.

During follow-up, patients with type 2 HRS may develop type 1 HRS, either spontaneously or due to the presence of a precipitating factor, usually an associated bacterial infection [20–22].

9.1.1. Differential diagnosis

The diagnosis of HRS involves excluding other causes for the development of renal failure in a cirrhotic patient, since they can present different causes, such as hypovolaemia, bacterial infections, acute tubular necrosis, administration of nephrotoxic drugs (non-steroidal anti-inflammatory drugs, antibiotics such as gentamicin, etc.) and parenchymal nephropathy.

There are no objective variables by which these causes of renal failure can be distinguished, which sometimes make differential diagnosis complicated, especially when trying to discriminate between HRS and acute tubular necrosis. Their diagnostic criteria are described subsequently [23, 24] (**Table 5**).

- Presence of cirrhosis with ascites
- Serum creatinine >1.5 mg/dl
- No improvement in serum creatinine levels, at least 2 days after discontinuing diuretics and then expanding the blood volume by infusions of albumin at a dose of 1 g/kg of body weight/day, up to a maximum of 100 g/day
- Absence of shock
- No evidence of recent intake of nephrotoxic drugs
- Absence of renal parenchymal disease as evidenced by the presence of proteinuria (>500 mg/day), microhaematuria (>50 red cells/high-magnification field) and/or an abnormal renal ultrasound result.

Table 5. Diagnostic criteria for hepatorenal syndrome.

9.2. Treatment

HRS treatment depends on the severity of renal failure and its associated complications. Patients with type 1 HRS who are on a liver transplant waiting list should be treated in an intensive or intermediate care unit, with close monitoring to detect any intercurrent complications at an early stage.

By contrast, patients with type 2 HRS without associated complications can be controlled on an outpatient basis. Therefore, we describe the therapeutic options available to patients with type 1 HRS.

9.2.1. Vasoconstrictors

The use of vasoconstrictors in conjunction with the intravenous administration of albumin is considered the first-line treatment in the management of patients with type 1 HRS.

Vasoconstrictors used include vasopressin analogues, especially terlipressin and alpha-adrenergic agonists, such as noradrenaline and midodrine.

Treatment with terlipressin and albumin produces a significant improvement in renal function in 40–50% of patients and is accompanied by improved survival.

Treatment usually starts at a dose of 1 mg/4 h in the form of intravenous boluses, increasing to 2 mg/4 h after 3 days if there is no response (defined as a decrease in creatinine by more than 25% of the baseline level).

Relapse after treatment is infrequent; if it occurs, it is advisable to repeat the same treatment [25–27].

Patients being treated with vasoconstrictors and albumin should be monitored closely in order to detect the presence of possible side effects. These are mainly of an ischaemic and cardiovascular nature and can appear in 10–15% of cases. The treatment is also effective and safe in patients with associated bacterial infections.

9.2.2. Other vasoconstrictors

The wider availability and lower cost of noradrenaline and midodrine, both in combination with albumin, make them an attractive alternative to treatment with terlipressin. The efficacy and safety of noradrenaline are similar to those of terlipressin in the treatment of patients with type 1 HRS. The same is true of midodrine, although clinical experience of its use is more limited.

Norepinephrine is given at a dose of 0.5–3.0 mg/h in continuous intravenous infusion, with the aim of increasing the mean blood pressure to 10 mm Hg. Treatment is continued until the level of blood creatinine drops below 1.5 mg/dl.

9.2.3. TIPS

TIPS may be considered an alternative treatment to that with vasoconstrictors, since it also improves renal function in this type of patient. Its clinical application under these circumstances is rather limited, since many patients with type 1 HRS present contraindications for its implementation, of which the most frequent and serious is advanced liver failure.

9.2.4. Renal substitution therapy (hepatic dialysis)

This treatment modality is only indicated in patients with type 1 HRS who do not respond to treatment with vasoconstrictors and albumin, and who develop criteria requiring urgent dialysis, such as hypervolaemia, hyperkalaemia, metabolic acidosis, and so on. Fortunately, however, these situations are rare in this group of patients.

Other dialysis methods include the use of the molecular adsorbent recirculation system (MARS) and Prometheus, a dialysis machine to which a module is added for fractional plasma separation and adsorption. However, their usefulness is very limited in these patients.

9.2.5. Liver transplant

Liver transplant is the definitive treatment and therefore the first choice for patients with types 1 and 2 HRS. Therefore, every patient who presents an HRS should be referred to a reference centre where the operation can be performed.

Its functional nature makes HRS potentially reversible after orthotopic liver transplantation (OLT) without associated renal transplantation. Double transplantation (liver and kidney) should only be considered in patients who have required prolonged renal support for 6–8 weeks, because the probability of their HRS reverting is very low.

Patients with type 1 HRS should be prioritized on the transplant waiting list, since they are at a high risk of early mortality. The use of the model for end-stage liver disease (MELD) scoring method as an organ distribution system has made it possible to prioritize these patients, since it includes serum creatinine in the scoring.

It should be noted that although the renal function of patients with type 1 HRS improves after treatment with vasoconstrictors, the creatinine used to calculate the MELD score in these patients should be that obtained beforehand, at the beginning of treatment, so that they remain as priorities in the waiting list [28].

Treatment with vasoconstrictors and albumin before the liver transplant is recommended, since prior improvement of renal function may improve the prognosis during the post-transplant period.

Author details

Luis Rodrigo

Address all correspondence to: lrodrigosaez@gmail.com

University of Oviedo, Spain

References

[1] Garcia-Tsao G. Current management of the complications of cirrhosis and portal hypertension: Variceal hemorrhage, ascites and spontaneous bacterial peritonitis. Digestive Diseases. 2016;**34**:382-386

[2] Fukui H, Saito H, Ueno Y, Uto H, Obara K, Sakaida I, et al. Evidence-based clinical practice guidelines for liver cirrhosis 2015. Journal of Gastroenterology. 2016;**51**:629-650

[3] James J, Liou IW. Comprehensive care of patients with chronic liver disease. Medical Clinics of North America. 2015;**99**:913-933

[4] Pedersen JS, Bendtsen F, Møller S. Management of cirrhotic ascites. Therapeutic Advances in Chronic Disease. 2015;**6**:124-137

[5] Solá E, Solé C, Ginés P. Management of uninfected and infected ascites in cirrhosis. Liver International. 2016;**36**(Suppl 1):109-115

[6] Annamalai A, Wisdom L, Herada M, Nourredin M, Ayoub W, Sundaram V, et al. Management of refractory ascites in cirrhosis: Are we out of date? World Journal of Hepatology. 2016;**8**:1182-1193

[7] Sen Sarma M, Yachha SK, Bhatia V, Srivastava A, Poddar U. Safety, complications and outcome of large volume paracentesis with or without albumin therapy in children with severe ascites due to liver disease. Journal of Hepatology. 2015;**63**:1126-1132

[8] Sankar K, Moore CM. Transjugular intrahepatic portosystemic shunts. Journal of American Medical Association. 2017;**317**:880

[9] Sinha VK, Ko B. Hyponatremia in cirrhosis, pathogenesis, treatment and prognostic significance. Advances in Chronic Kidney Disease. 2015;**22**:361-367

[10] John S, Thuluvath PJ. Hyponatremia in cirrhosis: Pathophysiology and management. World Journal of Gastroenterology. 2015;**21**:3197-3205

[11] Bernardi M, Ricci CS, Santi L. Hyponatremia in patients with cirrhosis of the liver. Journal of Clinical Medicine. 2014;**4**:85-101

[12] Ginés P, Guevara M. Hyponatremia in cirrhosis: Pathogenesis, clinical significance and management. Hepatology 2008;**48**:1002-1010

[13] Lizaola B, Bonder A, Tapper EB, Mendez-Bocanegra A, Cardenas A. The changing role of sodium management in cirrhosis. Current Treatment Options in Gastroenterology. 2016;**14**:274-284

[14] Fukui H. Do vasopressin V2 receptor antagonists benefit cirrhotics with refractory ascites? World Journal of Gastroenterology. 2015;**21**:11584-11596

[15] Sakaida I, Terai S, Nakajima K, Shibasaki Y, Tachikawa S, Tsubouchi H. Predictive factors of the pharmacological action of tolvaptan in patients with liver cirrhosis: A post hoc analysis. Journal of Gastroenterology. 2017;**52**:229-236

[16] Dever JB, Sheikh MY. Spontaneous bacterial peritonitis-bacteriology, diagnosis, treatment, risk factors and prevention. Alimentary Pharmacology & Therapeutics. 2015;**41**: 1116-1131

[17] Piano S, Fasolato S, Salinas F, Romano A, Tonon M, Morando F, et al. The empirical antibiotic treatment of nosocomial spontaneous bacterial peritonitis: Results of a randomized, controlled clinical trial. Hepatology. 2016;**63**:1299-1309

[18] Ra G, Tsien C, Renner EL, Wong FS. The negative prognostic impact of a first episode of spontaneous bacterial peritonitis in cirrhosis and ascites. Journal of Clinical Gastroenterology. 2015;**49**:858-865

[19] Assem M, Elsabaawy M, Abdelrashed M, Elemam S, Khodeer S, Hamed W, et al. Efficacy and safety of alternating norfloxacin and rifaximin as primary prophylaxis for spontaneous bacterial peritonitis in cirrhotic ascites: A prospective randomized open-label comparative multicenter study. Hepatology International. 2016;**10**:377-385

[20] Angeli P, Gines P, Wong F, Bernardi M, Boyer TD, Gerbes A et al. International Club of Ascites. Diagnosis and management of acute kidney injury in patients with cirrhosis: Revised consensus recommendations of the International Club of Ascites. Gut. 2015;**64**:531-537

[21] Fabrizi F, Messa P. Challenges in renal failure treatment before liver transplant. Clinical Liver Disease. 2017;**21**:303-319

[22] Russ KB, Stevens TM, Singal AK. Acute kidney injury in patients with cirrhosis. Journal of Clinical and Translational Hepatology. 2015;**3**:195-204

[23] De Mattos ÁZ, De Mattos AA, Méndez-Sánchez N. Hepatorenal syndrome: Current concepts related to diagnosis and management. Annals of Hepatology. 2016;**15**:474-481

[24] Acevedo JG, Cramp ME. Hepatorenal syndrome: Update on diagnosis and therapy. World Journal of Hepatology. 2017;**9**:293-299

[25] Sanyal A, Boyer T, Garcia-Tsao G, Regenstein F, Rossaro L, Appenrodt B, et al. A prospective, randomized, double-blind, placebo-controlled trial of terlipressin for type 1 hepatorenal syndrome (HRS). Gastroenterology. 2008;**134**:1360-1368

[26] Martin-Llahi M, Pepin MN, Guevara G, Díaz F, Torre A, Monescillo A, et al. Terlipressin and albumin vs albumin in patients with cirrhosis and hepatorenal syndrome: A randomized study. Gastroenterology. 2008;**134**:1352-1359

[27] Boyer TD, Sanyal AJ, Wong F, Frederick RT, Lake JR, O'Leary JG, et al.; Reverse Study Investigators. Terlipressin plus albumin is more effective than albumin alone in improving renal function in patients with cirrhosis and hepatorenal syndrome type 1. Gastroenterology. 2016;**150**:1579-1589

[28] Ginés P, Fernández J, Durand F, Saliba F. Management of critically-ill cirrhotic patients. Journal of Hepatology. 2012;**56**(Suppl 1):S13-S24

Chapter 2

Cirrhotic Ascites: Pathophysiological Changes and Clinical Implications

Abdulrahman Bendahmash, Hussien Elsiesy and
Waleed K. Al-hamoudi

Additional information is available at the end of the chapter

http://dx.doi.org/10.5772/intechopen.70537

Abstract

Liver cirrhosis is associated with a wide range of systemic and pulmonary vascular abnormalities. Cardiac dysfunction also occurs in patients with advanced liver disease (cirrhotic cardiomyopathy). The circulation in cirrhosis is hyperdynamic, which is typically characterized by hypotension resulting from the associated vasodilatation and reflex tachycardia. The circulatory dysfunction in cirrhosis is the proposed pathophysiological mechanism leading to sodium and water retention in patients with liver cirrhosis. Hyperdynamic circulation is triggered by increased intrahepatic resistance due to cirrhosis, leading to a progressive increase in portal venous pressure. As portal hypertension worsens, local production of vasodilators increases due to endothelial activation, leading to splanchnic and systemic arterial vasodilation. Nitric oxide (NO) is considered one of the most important vasodilator molecules in the splanchnic and systemic circulation. The reduction in the effective arterial blood volume results in diminished renal arterial blood flow and subsequently triggers the rennin-angiotensin-aldosterone system (RAAS), antidiuretic hormones (ADHs) and sympathetic nervous system (SNS), leading to renal artery vasoconstriction. All these changes lead to sodium retention and volume expansion, manifested as ascites and peripheral edema. Furthermore, disease progression is associated with various degrees of renal dysfunction.

Keywords: cirrhosis, portal hypertension, hyperdynamic circulation, ascites

1. Introduction

Liver cirrhosis is associated with a wide range of systemic and pulmonary vascular abnormalities. Cardiac dysfunction has also been described in patients with advanced liver disease (cirrhotic cardiomyopathy) [1–4]. The circulation in cirrhosis has been described as being hyperdynamic, which is typically characterized by hypotension resulting from the associated vasodilatation and reflex tachycardia. These cardiovascular abnormalities play a major role in the pathogenesis of multiple life-threatening complications, including ascites, spontaneous bacterial peritonitis, hepatorenal syndrome (HRS), esophageal varices and pulmonary related complications [5, 6]. The hyperdynamic circulation is triggered by increased intrahepatic resistance due to cirrhosis, leading to a progressive increase in portal venous pressure [7, 8]. As portal hypertension worsens, there is an increased local production of vasodilators due to endothelial activation, leading to splanchnic and systemic arterial vasodilation. Nitric oxide (NO) is thought to be one of the most important vasodilator molecules in the splanchnic and systemic circulation. NO is overproduced in cirrhosis; measured serum levels are significantly elevated in both cirrhotic patients and in animal models [9–11]. The reduction in the effective arterial blood volume results in diminished renal arterial blood flow and subsequently triggers the rennin-angiotensin-aldosterone system (RAAS), antidiuretic hormone (ADH) and sympathetic nervous system (SNS), leading to renal artery vasoconstriction. All these changes lead to sodium retention and volume expansion, manifested as ascites and peripheral edema. Furthermore, advanced liver disease is usually associated with various degrees of renal dysfunction. In cirrhotic patients with hepatorenal syndrome (HRS), renal plasma flow and glomerular filtration rate (GFR) are significantly diminished and may reach levels similar to those seen in patients with advanced renal disease [12, 13]. Sodium retention usually occurs in association with the inability to excrete a normal water load, resulting in increased total body water and dilutional hyponatremia [14, 15]. However, unlike the situation of end-stage renal disease, no significant histological abnormality is present within the kidneys of patients with HRS, and the process is reversible after liver transplantation (LT) [16]. The aim of this chapter is to discuss the impact of portal hypertension on the cardiovascular system in cirrhosis, with special emphasis on the pathogenesis of ascites.

2. Ascites

The peritoneum is a serous membrane made up of visceral and parietal layers. The parietal peritoneum lines the coelomic cavity, and the visceral layer of the peritoneum lines the surface of organs. The peritoneal cavity is an empty space between the visceral and parietal layers of the peritoneum. The potential space of the peritoneal cavity is normally not visible on imaging as it contains only a small amount of fluid (approximately 100 mL). The fluid is mostly water with electrolytes, antibodies, white blood cells, albumin, glucose and other biochemicals [17]. Its main function is to reduce the friction between the abdominal organs as they move around during digestion. The word ascites is derived from the Greek word "askos," which means a bag or sack and is defined as pathological fluid accumulation within the peritoneal cavity. Ascites is a frequent complication of cirrhosis and portal hypertension because of the increase of the sinusoidal hydrostatic pressure. Cirrhosis accounts for over 75% of episodes of ascites, with all other causes accounting for less than 25% (**Table 1**) [18]. Ascites has been associated with increased morbidity and mortality, with liver transplant-free mortality rates ranging from 15 to 20% at 1 year to nearly 50–60% at 5 years from the time of diagnosis [19, 20].

http://dx.doi.org/10.5772/intechopen.70537

Causes of ascites
Portal hypertension
Infection
Heart failure
Malignancy and hematological disorders
Connective tissue disease
Pancreatic disease
Nephrotic syndrome
Severe malnutrition
Congenital causes

Table 1. Causes of ascites.

3. The heart (cirrhotic cardiomyopathy)

In 1953, Kowalski and Abelmann described an abnormal circulatory pattern in a group of cirrhotic patients. The examined the circulation in 22 alcoholic cirrhotic patients and concluded that these patients had a large stroke volume, prolonged Q-T interval and reduced peripheral vascular resistance. They were some of the first researchers to question the impact of liver disease on the heart [21]. These findings were then confirmed in multiple experimental models of portal hypertension and in patients with cirrhosis. Initially, it was thought that these circulatory manifestations were secondary to alcoholic-related malnutrition; however, future studies confirmed the same circulatory dysregulation in cirrhotic patients with various underlying etiologies [1–4]. In the absence of known cardiac disease, the diagnostic criteria for cirrhotic cardiomyopathy rest on the presence of an attenuated systolic or diastolic response to stressful stimuli and are supported by the presence of structural or histological changes in cardiac chambers, electrophysiological abnormalities and elevation in serum markers suggestive of cardiac stress [22]. In addition to abnormal systolic dysfunction, cirrhotic patients also clearly demonstrate abnormal diastolic dysfunction, especially in patients with ascites, and it has been shown that paracentesis can improve diastolic dysfunction. Left ventricular (LV) diastolic dysfunction manifests as impaired LV relaxation secondary to LV wall stiffness, which results in the increase in filling pressure. Glenn et al. investigated the role of passive tension regulators—titin and collagen—in the pathogenesis of cirrhotic diastolic dysfunction. They showed that alterations in titin modulation, PKA levels, and collagen configuration contributed to the pathogenesis of this condition [23]. Velocity of blood flow from the left atrium to the left ventricle during early (E wave) and late (A wave) phases of diastole can help in assessing diastolic function. A low E/A ratio indicates a non-compliant ventricle [24]. This finding was also confirmed in other studies [25, 26]. Multiple factors affecting cardiac cell function have been implicated in the pathogenesis of cirrhotic cardiomyopathy, including: (a) Down regulation of β-adrenergic receptors, which negatively impacts cardiac contractility [27]; (b) Reduction in the cardiac cell membrane fluidity, which impairs the function of membrane-bound ion channels, alters control of vascular tone and reduces the β-adrenoceptor function [28, 29]; (c) Reduced muscarinic receptor activity, which has a negative inotropic effect on the heart [30]; (d) Augmented nitric oxide activity, which negatively impacts cardiac contractility [31, 32]; (e) Carbon monoxide (CO) and endocannabinoid activity negatively impacts cardiac contractility in cirrhotic patients [33–35]. Multiple other studies have demonstrated significant structural cardiac abnormalities in all cardiac chambers of cirrhotic patients [36].

4. Systemic and splanchnic circulation

Portosystemic collaterals are formed secondary to cirrhosis-induced portal hypertension, which allows gut-derived humoral substances to directly enter systemic circulation without detoxification by the liver. Arterial vasodilatation in portal hypertension results from the predominant production of various vasodilators [37]. NO is thought to be the major vasodilator molecule in cirrhotic patients. The intrahepatic microcirculation is altered significantly in liver cirrhosis, secondary to both architectural and vasoactive humoral changes, resulting in an increase in vasoactive molecules associated with a decrease in intrahepatic NO production [38, 39]. On the other hand, multiple studies have documented an elevated serum level of NO in the systemic and splanchnic circulation in both cirrhotic patients and in animal models [40–43]. NO is an endothelial-derived relaxing factor that leads to systemic arterial vasodilatation. Three isoforms of NO synthase (NOS) have been described: endothelial (eNOS), inducible (iNOS), and neuronal (nNOS). However, the leading isoform contributing to these vascular changes remains obscure [44]. Ferguson and colleagues were the first group to use a highly selective iNOS inhibitor to evaluate the role iNOS in the regulation of vascular tone in patients with ascites. Forearm blood flow was measured in eight patients with ascites and was compared with eight matched healthy volunteers, during intrabrachial infusion of 1400 W (0.1–1 μmol/min), NG-monomethyl-L-arginine (L-NMMA, a non-selective NOS inhibitor; 2–8 μmol), and norepinephrine. They showed that iNOS inhibitor causes systemic vasoconstriction in patients with ascites only. This supports the role of iNOS in the circulatory changes associated with cirrhosis [45]. One major factor that plays an important role in promoting NO production is the altered intestinal permeability in patients with advanced liver disease. As a result various endotoxins cross the intestine to the systemic circulation and stimulate the production of NO [46, 47]. TNF-α is also considered to be a NO inducers. Inhibition of TNF-α production resulted in improvement in the hyperdynamic circulation in various animal model studies [48, 49]. Endocannabinoids have also been implicated in the peripheral vasodilatation of cirrhosis. Activation of endothelial cannabinoid receptors by the endogenously produced endocannabinoids causes pronounced vasodilatation in cirrhotic rats [50, 51]. Interestingly, multiple studies have shown a potentially important role of the central nervous system (CNS) in the pathogenesis of the portal hypertension-induced hyperdynamic circulation. The cardiovascular system is controlled by neural influences that include the central nervous system (CNS) and peripheral afferent and efferent nerves. Portal hypertension activates receptors in the mesenteric area; the signals are relayed to central

Pathogenic mechanisms	Cardiovascular effect
Down regulation of β-adrenergic receptors	Decreases cardiac contractility
Reduction in the cardiac cell membrane fluidity	Alters control of vascular tone and reduces the β-adrenoceptor function
Reduced muscarinic receptor activity	Negative inotropic effect on the heart
Augmented nitric oxide activity	Decreases cardiac contractility
Carbon monoxide	Decreases cardiac contractility
Endocannabinoid activity	Decreases cardiac contractility
Portosystemic collaterals	This allows gut-derived humoral substances to directly enter the systemic circulation augmenting the hyperdynamic circulation
Systemic nitric oxide	Systemic vasodilatation
Central nervous system-gut-axis	Denervation prevents the development of hyperdynamic circulation and ascites formation
Activation of renin-angiotensin aldosterone system, sympathetic nervous system and nonosmotic release of antidiuretic hormone	Restores the normal hemodynamics in the setting of a hyperdynamic circulation through sodium and water retention

Table 2. Pathogenic mechanisms of cardiovascular disturbance in cirrhotic patients.

cardiovascular-regulatory nuclei via afferent nerves. These nuclei then process the inputs and send out signals to the cardiovascular system through efferent pathways, leading to cardiovascular changes [52]. Li and colleagues demonstrated that neonatal capsaicin denervation in rats prevented the development of hyperdynamic circulation and renal dysfunction as well as ascites formation in cirrhosis. These results indicate that intact primary afferent innervation is necessary for the development of hyperdynamic circulation and ascites formation [53]. A recent study revealed reversal of the cirrhosis associated vascular dysregulation after afferent denervation in an animal model. Portal vein ligation in cirrhotic rats activates a marker protein in the brain stem indicating CNS activation. Furthermore, blocking CNS Fos expression in cirrhotic rats resulted in eliminating the development of the hyperdynamic circulation [54]. The various potential pathogenic mechanisms leading to cardiovascular disturbance and fluid retention are summarized in **Table 2**.

5. The lymphatic system

The lymphatic vascular system plays a critical role in ascites formation [55]. Lymphatic vessels remove fluid from the interstitial fluid from various parts of the body and drain it into the blood stream. In healthy adult individuals, the lymphatic system returns as much as eight liters of interstitial fluid with 20–30 g of protein per liter to venous circulation every day. Any disturbance to this process leads to fluid accumulation, manifested as edema and ascites [55–58]. As with systemic and splanchnic circulation, the lymphatic system is also influenced by nitric oxide, leading to vasodilatation [59]. The development of portal hypertension in cirrhosis is associated with an increase in portal lymph flow. Normally, the liver produces a large amount of lymph, which is estimated to be over 25% of the lymph flowing through the thoracic duct. Barrowman and colleagues demonstrated an increase in lymph flows from the intestine and liver in cirrhotic animals by threefold and 30-fold, respectively, over values obtained from control animals. They also demonstrated a good correlation between intestinal and liver lymph flows and portal venous pressure [60]. In portal hypertension, compensatory lymphangiogenic response may initially help to reduce the high portal pressure. Oikawa and colleagues used a morphometric analysis to examine portal hypertensive-associated changes in lymph vessels and branches of the portal vein, with use of immunohistochemical staining for alpha smooth muscle actin, and quantitated these changes using an image analysis system. They obtained wedge liver biopsies from 10 patients with advanced portal hypertension and 10 control samples from patients with gastric carcinoma without liver disease. They showed that the proliferation of lymph vessels were higher in portal hypertension samples compared to the control samples. On the other hand, the number of portal vein branches in portal hypertension samples was not different from control samples. They concluded that these alterations in portal hypertension may result in a decrease in portal flow associated with an increase in lymph flow resulting in a reduction of the high portal vein pressure in idiopathic portal hypertension [61]. With worsening liver fibrosis and ongoing portal hypertension, the lymphatic system fails, resulting in buildup of interstitial fluids and ascites formation [55].

6. Renal response

The systemic vasodilation in patients with cirrhosis leads to under filling of arterial vascular space and that leads to systemic hypotension. Consequently, baroreceptor-mediated activation of the renin-angiotensin-aldosterone system (RAAS) and sympathetic nervous system (SNS) and nonosmotic release of antidiuretic hormone (ADH) occur to restore normal hemodynamics. This leads to fluid and sodium retention (**Figure 1**). Sodium retention is the most common abnormality of renal function in patients with cirrhosis and ascites [12, 62, 63]. The total amount of sodium retained in patients with cirrhosis is dependent on sodium intake, non-renal sodium losses and sodium excreted in the urine. Minimizing sodium intake in cirrhotic patients may help control ascites. With ongoing hemodynamic disturbance in cirrhosis, the equation tips toward sodium retention. Associated with this is an increase in splanchnic permeability that, aided by the changes in oncotic pressure, combines to lead to ascites formation [63]. In the initial phases of the disease, this is compensated by an increase in lymph return. In fact, the thoracic duct lymph flow, which in normal conditions is lower than 1 liter per day, may increase by several folds. When lymph formation overcomes lymph drainage, this also results in ascites formation. As a result, renal vasoconstriction persists and results in various degrees of renal impairment. The extreme effect would result in severe renal failure with elevation of blood urea nitrogen and serum-creatinine concentration. The associated hyponatremia in portal hypertensive ascites carries a bad prognostic value and has been linked to mortality [64].

Refractory ascites refers to ascites that cannot be resolved by dietary sodium restriction and diuretic treatment. The severity of renal sodium retention increases with the progression of

http://dx.doi.org/10.5772/intechopen.70537

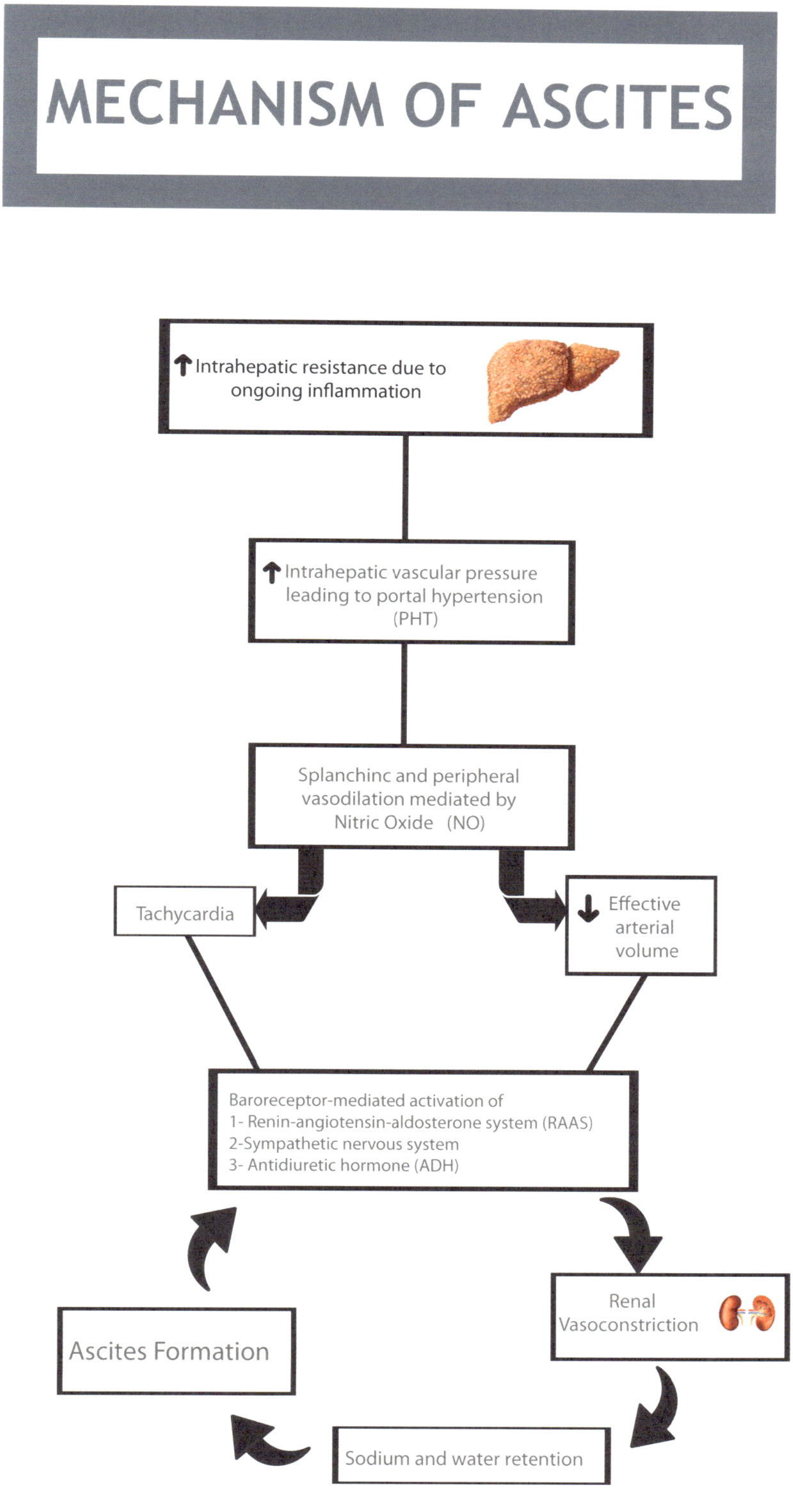

Figure 1. The cascade of changes leading to ascites formation.

the underlying liver disease and associated portal and systemic hemodynamic disturbance. The ongoing activation of the various neurohumoral pathways leads to aggressive renal reabsorption of sodium and water. Activation of the neurhormonal pathway also leads to a reduction in the glomerular filtration rate (GFR) and subsequently leads to a decline in the renal function. The enhanced sodium reabsorption at the proximal convoluted tubule leads to a significant reduction in the sodium reaching the distal segments of the nephron. This explains the failure of loop diuretics and antimineralocorticoid in treating these patients as they work predominantly at the distal segments of the nephron. Thus, renal sodium retention mainly occurs proximally to the site of action of both antimineralocorticoid and loop diuretics, and this can explain why diuretic treatment becomes unsuccessful in some patients. Furthermore, when cirrhosis progresses and the arterial vasodilation becomes more marked, the heart can no longer keep pace with the marked systemic vasodilatation. This results in an increase in the production of endogenous vasoactive compounds, which further increases sodium and water retention as a result of this physiological response to the relative arterial underfilling [63, 64]. This increased sodium and water retention contributes to increasing ascites, and in many cases, to the development of refractory ascites and type 2 HRS. Kraq and colleagues investigated the relation between cardiac and renal function in patients with cirrhosis and ascites and the impact of cardiac systolic function on survival. Cardiac function was investigated by gated myocardial perfusion imaging for assessment of cardiac index and cardiac volumes. Renal function was assessed by determination of GFR and renal blood flow, and the patients were followed up for 12 months. They demonstrated that patients with a low CI had a lower GFR and a higher creatinine level. The number of patients who developed type 1 HRS within 3 months was significantly higher in the group with low CI than that in the group with high CI. They also showed that patients with the lowest CI had significantly poorer survival at 3, 9, and 12 months than did those with a higher CI [65].

7. Clinical implications

This circulatory dysfunction in cirrhosis is the proposed pathophysiological mechanism leading to sodium and water retention in patients with liver cirrhosis. Treatment aimed at reversing this pathophysiological process would likely result in improving the outcome. Albumin has been used in clinical trials as a volume expander and, when given with a vasoconstrictor, has been shown to improve renal function in the setting of cirrhotic ascites. Martín-Llahí and colleagues randomized 46 patients with cirrhosis and HRS to receive terlipressin, a vasopressin analog, and albumin (n = 23) or albumin alone (n = 23) for a maximum of 15 days. They monitored renal function closely during the study period. Improvement of renal function occurred in 10 patients (43.5%) treated with terlipressin and albumin compared with that in two patients (8.7%) treated with albumin alone (P = .017) [66]. Similarly, Guevara and colleagues treated 16 patients with HRS with a combination of ornipressin, a potent vasoconstrictor agent, and albumin to improve the cardiovascular dysfunction. The combined treatment was administered for either 3 or 15 days (eight patients each). The shorter treatment duration was associated with normalization of the overactivity of renin-angiotensin and sympathetic nervous systems, a marked increase in atrial-natriuretic peptide levels, and only a slight improvement in renal function. However, when treatment was administered for 15 days outcome was significantly better. Renal function improved dramatically manifested by normalization of serum creatinine associated with an increase in the GFR and a persistent suppression in the activity of vasoconstrictor systems [67]. In another study, Ortega and colleagues showed that terlipressin therapy reverses HRS, and the effect was augmented when coupled with albumin [68]. Patel and colleagues assessed the efficacy of midodrine and octreotide as a therapeutic approach to increasing urinary electrolyte-free water clearance in advanced cirrhosis. Patients were treated with albumin, midodrine and octreotide within the first 24 h. Urinary electrolyte-free water clearance and serum sodium concentration were assessed before and 72 h after treatment. The assessments showed a statistically significant increase in serum sodium concentration and urinary electrolyte-free water clearance with the use of midodrine and octreotide in the treatment of cirrhosis-associated hyponatremia [69]. These studies demonstrate the importance of targeting circulatory dysfunction in end-stage liver disease. A more challenging aspect in managing these patients is the associated cirrhotic cardiomyopathy. The development of HRS in the setting of advanced liver disease is associated with a drop in the cardiac output, emphasizing the additional role of cirrhotic cardiomyopathy in the pathogenesis of hepatorenal dysfunction [65]. Other reports suggested a possible role of cirrhotic cardiomyopathy in spontaneous bacterial peritonitis [70].

Transjugular intrahepatic portosystemic shunts (TIPS) have been commonly used to treat refractory ascites. Following TIPS insertion, a sudden increase in the preload results in further hemodynamic disturbance, and therefore, careful cardiovascular evaluation prior to the procedure is a necessity [71, 72]. The preexisting subclinical diastolic dysfunction becomes clinically obvious with the sudden increase in the right atrial and pulmonary circulation, leading to heart failure. In a recent study, Ascha and colleagues investigated if echocardiographic and hemodynamic changes at the time of TIPS can provide any prognostic information. After evaluating 418 patients, they showed that a change in the right atrial (RA) pressure after TIPS predicted long-term mortality [73]. Others showed a possible impact of intra-procedural RA pressure on early post-TIPS mortality [74]. Other studies suggested that an E/A ratio of ≤ 1 was predictive of slow ascites clearance and mortality post-TIPS insertion [75, 76].

Liver transplantation results in correction of portal hypertension and reversal of all the pathophysiological mechanisms that lead to hyperdynamic circulation [77]. We studied the hemodynamics in the immediate post-transplant period and compared patients with alcoholic vs. viral cirrhosis. Within the first 24 h, there was a significant decrease in HR and increase in MAP; the extent of the change was similar in both groups. The central venous pressure (CVP), pulmonary capillary wedge pressure (PCWP), and systemic vascular resistance index (SVRI) increased, and changes were more pronounced in the viral group [78]. Navasa and colleagues assessed systemic hemodynamics and plasma levels of aldosterone, glucagon and plasma renin in 12 patients with advanced cirrhosis before and 2 weeks and 2 months after LT. Elevated aldosterone, plasma renin and glucagon levels decreased to near-normal values 2 weeks after transplantation. This decrease was associated with reversal of the associated splanchnic and systemic vasodilation and restoration of normal hemodynamics [79]. Following LT, the rapid reversal of systemic vasodilatation and the associated increase in blood pressure exposes the previously subclinical cirrhotic cardiomyopathy. Cardiovascular complications are a major cause of postoperative morbidity and mortality after liver transplantation [80]. Fouad and colleagues reviewed 197 liver transplant recipients for post-liver transplant-related cardiac complications. Eighty-two patients suffered one or more cardiac complications within 6 months after LT. Pulmonary edema was the most common complication, occurring in 61 patients; other complications included heart failure (7 patients), arrhythmia (13 patients), pulmonary hypertension (7 patients), pericardial effusion (2 patients), and cardiac thrombus formation (1 patient). In their study, cardiac causes were the leading cause of death (23.8% of all mortality) [81].

LT induces significant cardiovascular stress. Predicting the development of postoperative cardiac complications is very difficult. Two-dimensional and dobutamine stress echocardiography were utilized to predict the development of adverse cardiac events following liver transplantation, and both had a low predictive value [82]. More recently, a study utilizing dobutamine stress perfusion, which provides an assessment of both regional systolic and diastolic function as well as microvascular perfusion, revealed a better prediction of post-transplant cardiac outcome [83]. Management at the time of liver transplantation should involve careful fluid management. Immediate postoperative care should include continuous cardiac and hemodynamic monitoring and early detection of any potential arrhythmia or any other cardiac complication.

Author details

Abdulrahman Bendahmash[1], Hussien Elsiesy[2,3] and Waleed K. Al-hamoudi[2,4*]

*Address all correspondence to: walhamoudi@gmail.com

1 Department of Pediatrics, King Faisal Specialist Hospital & Research Center, Riyadh, Saudi Arabia

2 Department of Liver Transplantation, King Faisal Specialist Hospital & Research Center, Riyadh, Saudi Arabia

3 Department of Medicine, Alfaisal University, Riyadh, Saudi Arabia

4 Department of Medicine, College of Medicine, King Saud University, Riyadh, Saudi Arabia

References

[1] Ma Z, Lee SS. Cirrhotic cardiomyopathy: Getting to the heart of the matter. Hepatology. 1996;**24**:451-459

[2] Møller S, Henriksen JH. Cirrhotic cardiomyopathy: A pathophysiological review of circulatory dysfunction in liver disease. Heart. 2002;**87**:9-15

[3] Al Hamoudi W, Lee SS. Cirrhotic cardiomyopathy. Annals of Hepatology. 2006 Jul-Sep; **5**(3):132-139

[4] Al-Hamoudi WK. Cardiovascular changes in cirrhosis: Pathogenesis and clinical implications. Saudi Journal of Gastroenterology. 2010 Jul-Sep;**16**(3):145-153

[5] Salerno F, Gerbes A, Wong F, et al. Diagnosis, prevention and treatment of hepatorenal syndrome in cirrhosis. Gut. 2007;**56**:1310-1318

[6] Arroyo V, Gines P, Gerbes AL, et al. Definition and diagnostic criteria of refractory ascites and hepatorenal syndrome in cirrhosis. International ascites Club Hepatology. 1996;**23**:164-176

[7] Gines P, Fernandez-Esparrach G, Arroyo V, et al. Pathogenesis of ascites in cirrhosis. Seminars in Liver Disease. 1997;**17**:175-189

[8] Arroyo V, Badalamenti S, Gines P. Pathogenesis of ascites in cirrhosis. Minerva Medica. 1987;**78**:645-650

[9] Chang SW, Ohara N. Chronic biliary obstruction induces pulmonary intravascular phagocytosis and endotoxin sensitivity in rats. The Journal of Clinical Investigation. 1994;**94**:2009-2019

[10] Carter EP, Hartsfield CL, Miyazono M, Jakkula M, Morris KG Jr, McMurtry IF. Regulation of heme oxygenase-1 by nitric oxide during hepatopulmonary syndrome. American Journal of Physiology. Lung Cellular and Molecular Physiology. 2002;**283**:L346-L353

[11] Sztrymf B, Rabiller A, Nunes H, Savale L, Lebrec D, Le Pape A, et al. Prevention of hepatopulmonary syndrome and hyperdynamic state by pentoxifylline in cirrhotic rats. The European Respiratory Journal. 2004;**23**:752-758

[12] Jalan R, Forrest EH, Redhead DN, et al. Reduction in renal blood flow following acute increase in the portal pressure: Evidence for the existence of a hepatorenal reflex in man? Gut. 1997;**40**:664-670

[13] Ming Z, Smyth DD, Lautt WW. Decreases in portal flow trigger a hepatorenal reflex to inhibit renal sodium and water excretion in rats: Role of adenosine. Hepatology. 2002;**35**:167-175

[14] Arroyo V, Claria J, Salo J, Jimnez W. Antidiuretic hormone and the pathogenesis of water retention in cirrhosis with ascites. Seminars in Liver Disease. 1994;**14**:44-58

[15] McCullough AJ, Mullen KD, Kalhan SC. Measurements of total body and extracellular water in cirrhotic patients with and without ascites. Hepatology. 1991;**14**:1102-1111

[16] Mindikoglu AL, Pappas SC. New developments in Hepatorenal syndrome. Clinical Gastroenterology and Hepatology. 2017 Jun 7; pii: S1542-3565(17)30672-9 [Epub ahead of print]

[17] Pannu H, Oliphant M. The subperitoneal space and peritoneal cavity: Basic concepts. Abdominal Imaging. 2015;**40**(7):2710-2722

[18] Reynolds TB. Ascites. Clinics in Liver Disease. 2000;**4**:151-168

[19] Planas R, Montoliu S, Ballesté B, et al. Natural history of patients hospitalized for management of cirrhotic ascites. Clinical Gastroenterology and Hepatology. 2006;**4**:1385-1394

[20] Heuman DM, Abou-Assi SG, Habib A, et al. Persistent ascites and low serum sodium identify patients with cirrhosis and low MELD scores who are at high risk for early death. Hepatology. 2004;**40**:802-810

[21] Kowalski HJ, Abelmann WH. The cardiac output at rest in Laennec's cirrhosis. The Journal of Clinical Investigation. 1953 Oct;**32**(10):1025-1033

[22] Yang YY, Lin HC. The heart: Pathophysiology and clinical implications of cirrhotic cardiomyopathy. Journal of the Chinese Medical Association. 2012;**75**:619-623

[23] Glenn TK, Honar H, Liu H, ter Keurs HE, Lee SS. Role of cardiac myofilament proteins titin and collagen in the pathogenesis of diastolic dysfunction in cirrhotic rats. Journal of Hepatology. 2011;**55**:1249-1255

[24] Lee RF, Glenn TK, Lee SS. Cardiac dysfunction in cirrhosis. Best Practice & Research. Clinical Gastroenterology. 2007;**21**:125-140

[25] Finucci G, Desideri A, Sacerdoti D, et al. Left ventricular diastolic function in liver cirrhosis. Scandinavian Journal of Gastroenterology. 1996;**31**(3):279-284

[26] Pozzi M, Carugo S, Boari G, et al. Evidence of functional and structural cardiac abnormalities in cirrhotic patients with and without ascites. Hepatology. 1997;**26**(5):1131-1137

[27] Lee SS, Marty J, Mantz J, Samain E, Braillon A, Lebrec D. Desensitization of myocardial β-adrenergic receptors in cirrhotic rats. Hepatology. 1990;**12**:481-485

[28] Ma Z, Lee SS, Meddings JB. Effects of altered cardiac membrane fluidity on beta -adrenergic receptor signalling in rats with cirrhoticcardiomyopathy. Journal of Hepatology. 1997;**26**:904-912

[29] Le Grimellec C, Friedlander G, el Yandouzi EH, Zlatkine P, Giocondi MC. Membrane fluidity and transport properties in epithelia. Kidney International 1992;**42**:825-836.

[30] Jaue DN, Ma Z, Lee SS. Cardiac muscarinic receptor function in rats with cirrhotic cardiomyopathy. Hepatology. 1997;**25**:1361-1365

[31] Balligand JL, Kelly RA, Marsden PA, Smith TW, Michel T. Control of cardiac muscle cell function by an endogenous nitric oxide signaling system. Proceedings of the National Academy of Sciences of the United States of America. 1993;**90**:347-351

[32] Liu H, Ma Z, Lee SS. Contribution of nitric oxide to the pathogenesis of cirrhotic cardiomyopathy in bile duct-ligated rats. Gastroenterology. 2000;**118**:937-944

[33] Liu H, Song D, Lee SS. Role of heme oxygenase - carbon monoxide pathway in pathogenesis of cirrhotic cardiomyopathy in the rat. American Journal of Physiology. Gastrointestinal and Liver Physiology. 2001;**280**:G68-G74

[34] Bonz A, Laser M, Küllmer S, Kniesch S, Babin-Ebell J, Popp V, et al. Cannabinoids acting on CB1 receptors decrease contractile performance in human atrial muscle. Journal of Cardiovascular Pharmacology. 2003;**41**:657-664

[35] Ford WR, Honan SA, White R, Hiley CR. Evidence of a novel site mediating anandamide-induced negative inotropic and coronary vasodilatator responses in rat isolated hearts. British Journal of Pharmacology. 2002;**135**:1191-1198

[36] Alqahtani SA, Fouad TR, Lee SS. Cirrhotic cardiomyopathy. Seminars in Liver Disease. 2008;**28**:59-69

[37] Kim MY, Baik SK, Lee SS. Hemodynamic alterations in cirrhosis and portal hypertension. The Korean Journal of Hepatology. 2010 Dec;**16**(4):347-352

[38] Sanyal AJ, Bosch J, Blei A, Arroyo V. Portal hypertension and its complications. Gastroenterology. 2008;**134**:1715-1728

[39] Hendrickson H, Chatterjee S, Cao S, Morales Ruiz M, Sessa WC, Shah V. Influence of caveolin on constitutively activated recombinant eNOS: Insights into eNOS dysfunction in BDL rat liver. American Journal of Physiology. Gastrointestinal and Liver Physiology. 2003;**285**:652-660

[40] Wiest R, Shah V, Sessa WC, Groszmann RJ. NO overproduction by eNOS precedes hyperdynamic splanchnic circulation in portal hypertensive rats. The American Journal of Physiology. 1999;**276**:G1043-G1051

[41] Vallance P, Moncada S. Hyperdynamic circulation in cirrhosis: A role for nitric oxide? Lancet. 1991;**337**:776-778

[42] Genesca J, Gonzalez A, Segura R, Catalan R, Marti R, Varela E, Cadelina G, Martinez M, Lopez Talavera JC, Esteban R, Groszmann RJ, Guardia J. Interleukin-6, nitric oxide, and the clinical and hemodynamic alterations of patients with liver cirrhosis. The American Journal of Gastroenterology. 1999;**94**:169-177

[43] Hori N, Wiest R, Groszmann RJ. Enhanced release of nitric oxide in response to changes in flow and shear stress in the superior mesenteric arteries of portal hypertensive rats. Hepatology. 1998;**28**:1467-1473

[44] Martell M, Coll M, Ezkurdia N, Raurell I, Genescà J. Physiopathology of splanchnic vasodilation in portal hypertension. World Journal of Hepatology. 2010 Jun 27;**2**(6):208-220

[45] Ferguson JW, Dover AR, Chia S, Cruden NL, Hayes PC, Newby DE. Inducible nitric oxide synthase activity contributes to the regulation of peripheral vascular tone in patients with cirrhosis and ascites. Gut. 2006;**55**:542-546

[46] Bode C, Kugler V, Bode JC. Endotoxemia in patients with alcoholic and non-alcoholic cirrhosis and in subjects with no evidence of chronic liver disease following acute alcohol excess. Journal of Hepatology. 1987;**4**:8-14

[47] García-Tsao G. Bacterial translocation: Cause or consequence of decompensation in cirrhosis? Journal of Hepatology. 2001;**34**:150-155

[48] Lopez-Talavera JC, Merrill WW, Groszmann RJ. Tumor necrosis factor alpha: A major contributor to the hyperdynamic circulation in prehepatic portal-hypertensive rats. Gastroenterology. 1995;**108**:761-767

[49] Lopez-Talavera JC, Cadelina G, Olchowski J, Merrill W, Groszmann RJ. Thalidomide inhibits tumor necrosis factor alpha, decreases nitric oxide synthesis, and ameliorates the hyperdynamic circulatory syndrome in portal-hypertensive rats. Hepatology. 1996;**23**:1616-1621

[50] Moezi L, Gaskari SA, Lee SS. Endocannabinoids and liver disease. V. Endocannabinoids as mediators of vascular and cardiac abnormalities in cirrhosis. American Journal of Physiology. Gastrointestinal and Liver Physiology. 2008;**295**:G649-G653

[51] Bátkai S, Járai Z, Wagner JA, Goparaju SK, Varga K, Liu J, et al. Endocannabinoids acting at vascular CB1 receptors mediate the vasodilated state in advanced liver cirrhosis. Nature Medicine. 2001;**7**:827-832

[52] Song D, Liu H, Sharkey KA, Lee SS. Hyperdynamic circulation in portalhypertensive rats is dependent on central c-fos gene expression. Hepatology. 2002;**35**:159-166

[53] Li Y, Song D, Zhang Y, Lee SS. Effect of neonatal capsaicin treatment on haemodynamics and renal function in cirrhotic rats. Gut. 2003;**52**:293-299

[54] Liu H, Schuelert N, McDougall JJ, Lee SS. Central neural activation of hyperdynamic circulation in portal hypertensive rats depends on vagal afferent nerves. Gut. 2008;**57**:966-973

[55] Chung C, Iwakiri Y. The lymphatic vascular system in liver diseases: Its role in ascites formation. Clinical and Molecular Hepatology. 2013 Jun;**19**(2):99-104

[56] Harvey NL, Oliver G. Choose your fate: Artery, vein or lymphatic vessel? Current Opinion in Genetics & Development. 2004;**14**:499-505

[57] Oliver G, Alitalo K. The lymphatic vasculature: Recent progress and paradigms. Annual Review of Cell and Developmental Biology. 2005;**21**:457-483

[58] Tammela T, Alitalo K. Lymphangiogenesis: Molecular mechanisms and future promise. Cell. 2010;**140**:460-476

[59] Hagendoorn J, Padera TP, Kashiwagi S, Isaka N, Noda F, Lin MI, et al. Endothelial nitric oxide synthase regulates microlymphatic flow via collecting lymphatics. Circulation Research. 2004;**95**:204-209

[60] Barrowman JA, Granger DN. Effects of experimental cirrhosis on splanchnic microvascular fluid and solute exchange in the rat. Gastroenterology. 1984;**87**:165-172

[61] Oikawa H, Masuda T, Sato S, Yashima A, Suzuki K, Sato S, et al. Changes in lymph vessels and portal veins in the portal tract of patients with idiopathic portal hypertension: A morphometric study. Hepatology. 1998;**27**:1607-1610

[62] DiBona GF, Sawin LL. Hepatorenal baroreflex in cirrhotic rats. The American Journal of Physiology. 1995;**269**:29-33

[63] Fortune B, Cardenas A. Ascites, refractory ascites and hyponatremia in cirrhosis. Gastroenterology report (Oxford). 2017 May;**5**(2):104-112

[64] Salerno F, Guevara M, Bernardi M, Moreau R, Wong F, Angeli P, Garcia-Tsao G, Lee SS. Refractory ascites: Pathogenesis, definition and therapy of a severe complication in patients with cirrhosis. Liver International. 2010 Aug;**30**(7):937-947

[65] Krag A, Bendtsen F, Henriksen JH, et al. Low cardiac output predicts development of hepatorenal syndrome and survival in patients with cirrhosis and ascites. Gut. 2010;**59**:105-110

[66] Martín-Llahí M, Pépin MN, Guevara M, Díaz F, Torre A, Monescillo A, Soriano G, Terra C, Fábrega E, Arroyo V, Rodés J, Ginès P, TAHRS Investigators. Terlipressin and albumin vs albumin in patients with cirrhosis and hepatorenal syndrome: A randomized study. Gastroenterology. 2008 May;**134**(5):1352-1359

[67] Guevara M, Ginès P, Fernández-Esparrach G, Sort P, Salmerón JM, Jiménez W, Arroyo V, Rodés J. Reversibility of hepatorenal syndrome by prolonged administration of ornipressin and plasma volume expansion. Hepatology. 1998 Jan;**27**(1):35-41

[68] Ortega R, Ginès P, Uriz J, Cárdenas A, Calahorra B, De Las Heras D, Guevara M, Bataller R, Jiménez W, Arroyo V, Rodés J. Terlipressin therapy with and without albumin for patients with hepatorenal syndrome: Results of a prospective, nonrandomized study. Hepatology. 2002 Oct;**36**(4 Pt 1):941-948

[69] Patel S, Nguyen DS, Rastogi A, Nguyen MK, Nguyen MK. Treatment of cirrhosis-associated Hyponatremia with Midodrine and Octreotide. Frontiers in Medicine (Lausanne). 2017 Mar 14;**4**:17

[70] Lee SS. Cardiac dysfunction in spontaneous bacterial peritonitis: A manifestation of cirrhotic cardiomyopathy? Hepatology. 2003 Nov;**38**(5):1089-1091

[71] Azoulay D, Castaing D, Dennison A, Martino W, Eyraud D, Bismuth H. Transjugular intrahepatic portosystemic shunt worsen the hyperdynamic circulatory state of the cirrhotic patient: Preliminary report of a prospective study. Hepatology. 1994;**19**:129-132

[72] Rodríguez-Laiz JM, Bañares R, Echenagusia A, Casado M, Camuñez F, Pérez-Roldán F, et al. Effects of transjugular intrahepatic portasystemic shunt (TIPS) on splanchnic and systemic hemodynamics, and hepatic function in patients with portal hypertension. Preliminary results. Digestive Diseases and Sciences. 1995;**40**:2121-2127

[73] Ascha M, Abuqayyas S, Hanouneh I, Alkukhun L, Sands M, Dweik RA, Tonelli AR. Predictors of mortality after transjugular portosystemic shunt. World Journal of Hepatology. 2016 Apr 18;**8**(11):520-529

[74] Parvinian A, Bui JT, Knuttinen MG, Minocha J, Gaba RC. Right atrial pressure may impact early survival of patients undergoing transjugular intrahepatic portosystemic shunt creation. Annals of Hepatology. 2014 Jul-Aug;**13**(4):411-419

[75] Rabie RN, Cazzaniga M, Salerno F, Wong F. The use of E/A ratio as a predictor of outcome in cirrhotic patients treated with transjugular intrahepatic portosystemic shunt. The American Journal of Gastroenterology. 2009;**104**:2458-2466

[76] Cazzaniga M, Salerno F, Pagnozzi G, Dionigi E, Visentin S, Cirello I, et al. Diastolic dysfunction is associated with poor survival in cirrhotic patients with transjugular intrahepatic portosystemic shunt. Gut. 2007;**56**:869-875

[77] Liu H, Lee SS. What happens to cirrhotic cardiomyopathy after liver transplantation? Hepatology. 2005 Nov;**42**(5):1203-1205

[78] Al-Hamoudi WK, Alqahtani S, Tandon P, Ma M, Lee SS. Hemodynamics in the immediate post-transplantation period in alcoholic and viral cirrhosis. World Journal of Gastroenterology. 2010 Feb 7;**16**(5):608-612

[79] Navasa M, Feu F, García-Pagán JC, Jiménez W, Llach J, Rimola A, et al. Hemodynamic and humoral changes after liver transplantation in patients with cirrhosis. Hepatology. 1993;**17**:355-360

[80] Liu H, Jayakumar S, Traboulsi M, Lee SS. Cirrhotic cardiomyopathy: Implications for liver transplantation. Liver Transplantation. 2017 Jun;**23**(6):826-835

[81] Fouad TR, Abdel-Razek WM, Burak KW, Bain VG, Lee SS. Prediction of cardiac complications after liver transplantation. Transplantation. 2009;**87**:763-770

[82] Donovan CL, Marcovitz PA, Punch JD, Bach DS, Brown KA, Lucey MR, et al. Two-dimensional and dobutamine stress echocardiography in the preoperative assessment of patients with end-stage liver disease prior to orthotopic liver transplantation. Transplantation. 1996;**61**:1180-1188

[83] Baibhav B, Mahabir CA, Xie F, Shostrom VK, McCashland TM, Porter TR. Predictive value of Dobutamine stress perfusion echocardiography in contemporary end-stage liver disease. Journal of the American Heart Association. 2017 Feb 20;**6**(2). pii: e005102. [Epub ahead of print]

Chapter 3

Modern Tools for Diagnosis in Tuberculous Ascites

Andra-Iulia Suceveanu, Despina Todescu,
Laura Mazilu, Filippos Goniotakis Manousos,
Roxana Hulea, Felix Voinea, Eugen Dumitru and
Adrian Paul Suceveanu

Additional information is available at the end of the chapter

http://dx.doi.org/10.5772/intechopen.70417

Abstract

Tuberculosis (TB) is a highly contagious bacterial infection caused by *Mycobacterium tuberculosis* (MTB), affecting about 1/3rd of the world population and being responsible for lot of deaths worldwide, despite the progress achieved in the diagnosis and treatment fields. TB can affect the peritoneum, the TB ascites being a concern for physicians, especially when dealing with immunocompromised patients. The clinical presentation of TB ascites is challenging, due to nonspecific symptoms that make confusion with other diseases and the late results of cultures from ascites. The late diagnosis leads to a delayed treatment and high mortality. This manuscript describes recent tools used for early diagnosis in TB ascites. Molecular methods based on mycobacterial nucleic acid amplification tests (NAATs), polymerase chain reaction (PCR) detecting minimal amounts of bacterial DNA, or interferongamma release assays (IGRA) and biochemical methods such as the serum-ascites albumin gradient (SAAG) <1.1 g/dL, ratio between lactic dehydrogenase (LDH) in ascites fluid/serum total protein (TP) ratio of 0.5 and fluid ascites/serum LDH ratio of 0.6, and adenosine deaminase activity (ADA) > 40 UI/ml were recently considered more accurate diagnostic procedures. These methods allow a rapid and accurate differential diagnosis of ascites fluid, making possible the early treatment with appropriate drugs.

Keywords: peritoneal tuberculosis, ascites, diagnosis, molecular tests, biochemical tests

1. Introduction

Tuberculosis (TB) is a dangerous infection affecting about one third of the world population despite the availability of affordable and effective chemotherapy, remaining one of the major causes of death from a single infectious agent worldwide. The most affected organ is the lung. It is preventable through Bacillus of Calmette and Guérin (BCG) vaccination and curable with antituberculous drugs.

Tuberculosis is a serious and highly contagious bacterial infection which in humans is usually caused by bacteria called *Mycobacterium tuberculosis* (MTB), a member of the *Mycobacteriaceae* family. This complex also includes *M. bovis* and *M. africanum*. *M. bovis* is more frequently found in cattle and other animals, but it's also responsible for some cases in humans. *M. africanum* is more common in West African countries. Mycobacterial infection is spread through the air from one person to another and causes active disease or latent infection [1].

The absolute number of incident cases has been decreasing since the early 2000s. The lowest incidence rate is found in high-income countries including the United States of America, Canada, New Zealand, Western Europe, and Australia. The largest number of incident cases is found in low- and middle-income countries. In 2015, 61% of the new cases occurred in Asia, followed by 26% new cases in Africa (**Figure 1**) [2].

The HIV infection is the prevalent risk factor for the development of TB because HIV alters the pathogenesis of TB by producing a progressive decline in cell-mediated immunity and raises the chances of extrapulmonary involvement [3, 4].

Tuberculosis is a disease which typically involves the respiratory system, being characterized by the growth of tubercles in tissues, but it can affect any other organ, in which case it's called extrapulmonary tuberculosis (EPTB) and usually results from hematogenous dissemination, being particularly present in immunocompromised patients. In some cases the infection directly extends from an adjacent organ. The most common sites of extrapulmonary tuberculosis are the lymph nodes, abdomen, bones and joints, pleura, spinal cord, and brain [5, 6].

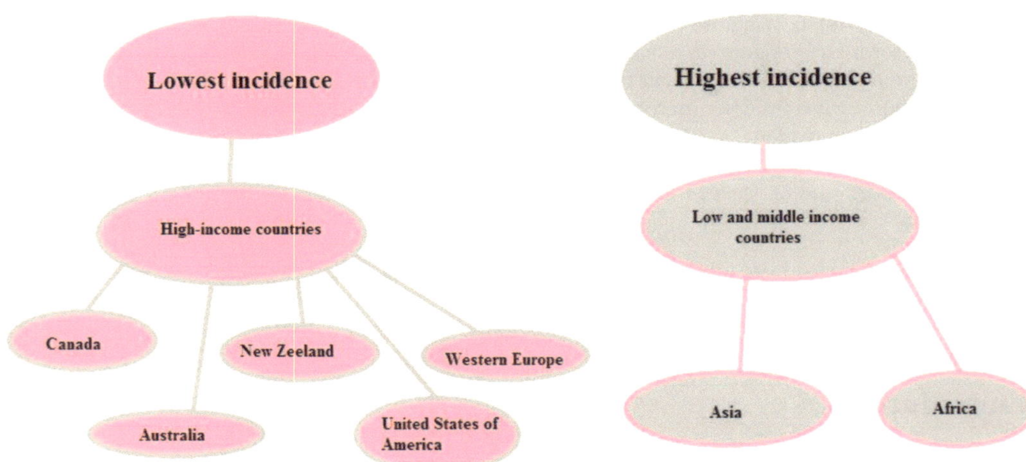

Figure 1. Worldwide incidence of TB infections.

http://dx.doi.org/10.5772/intechopen.70417

Abdominal tuberculosis is a common form of extrapulmonary tuberculosis. The infection involving *M. tuberculosis* or *M. bovis* could be the result of a primary infection or the reactivation of a latent focus in immunocompromised patients. The spread of abdominal tuberculosis can be hematogenous or can result from direct contact with primary focus or ingestion of sputum containing bacilli from the active pulmonary focus. This form of EPTB affects the peritoneum, the gut, the abdominal lymph nodes, and sometimes, less frequently, the parenchymatous organs in the abdomen like the spleen, liver, and pancreas leading to severe complications. There are three types of abdominal tuberculosis: ascitic, obstructive, and glandular. Diagnosis can be achieved through different methods: ultrasound of the abdomen, CT/MRI scans, biopsies of the suspected organ, endoscopy, and various function tests.

Peritoneal tuberculosis is an uncommon site of extrapulmonary infection caused by *M. tuberculosis*. Patients susceptible of developing EPTB are those with malignant diseases, HIV infection, diabetes, and cirrhosis or patients treated with antitumor necrosis factor (TNF) agents or peritoneal dialysis. Peritoneal TB is divided into three types: the wet ascitic type, the fixed fibrotic type, and the dry plastic type. The wet ascitic type is more common and is associated with large amounts of free or loculated fluid in the abdomen. The high attenuation of the ascites in abdominal ultrasound is thought to be due to high protein and cellular content. Associated peritoneal enhancement is usually present.

Infection occurs frequently following reactivation of latent tuberculous in the peritoneum from hematogenous spread from a primary lung focus. It can also occur via hematogenous spread from active pulmonary or miliary TB. Not so often, the organisms enter the peritoneal cavity transmurally, from an infected small intestine or contiguously from tuberculous salpingitis. Over time, the visceral and parietal peritoneum becomes studded with tubercles [7–9].

2. Definition

Ascites is defined as an abnormal accumulation of fluid in the peritoneal cavity, the presence of serous fluid between the visceral and parietal peritoneum. The word ascites is derived from the ancient Greek word "*askos*" meaning a bag or a sack. Under normal circumstances, the amount of peritoneal fluid depends on a balance between plasma flowing into and out of the blood and lymphatic vessels. This balance, once being disrupted, leads to abnormal accumulation of fluid [10]. Ascites can be a consequence or a complication of infections, malignancy, and many severe diseases: cardiac, endocrine, hepatic, or renal. The prognosis is usually poor, but it depends on the underlying causes. Laboratory tests of ascitic fluid, clinical, paraclinical, and pathological data are required for the differential diagnosis.

Tuberculous ascites, one of the clinical signs of abdominal TB, implies accumulation of fluid in the abdomen, a swollen abdomen, and slightly raised tubercles of 1–2 mm all over the peritoneum. In EPTB, ascites develops secondary to "exudation" of proteinaceous fluid from the tubercles, similar to the mechanism leading to ascites in patients with peritoneal carcinomatosis, and it's often misdiagnosed in elderly patients. Most patients with tuberculous peritonitis have ascites at the time of diagnosis, while the rest present the advanced phase, the dry or fibroadhesive form of the disease [11, 12].

3. Clinical manifestations

Tuberculous peritonitis is a subacute disease, and its symptoms evolve over a period of several weeks or months.

The insidious onset of this condition and the fact that the diagnosis is rarely suspected explains why patients have symptoms for more than 4 months before the diagnosis is established. Tuberculous peritonitis should be considered in any patient presenting with several weeks of abdominal pain, fever, and weight loss. Systemic and constitutional manifestations are common. Symptoms may be mild, with fatigue, abdominal pain, and tenderness, or severe enough to mimic acute abdomen [13]. Other clinical manifestations could be:

- Constipation/diarrhea
- Nocturnal hyperhidrosis
- Low-grade fever
- Anorexia
- Malaise

The clinical presentation of TB ascites is challenging, since it is nonspecific and can be confused with a plethora of other infectious or noninfectious diseases, leading to a delayed diagnosis and treatment which are major factors that contribute to the high mortality of TB.

Another situation that contributes to a delayed diagnosis is the presence of multiple comorbidities such as HIV/AIDS, cirrhosis, uremia, or other chronic conditions. Additional illness results in atypical presentation of TB ascites which render the symptoms more difficult to identify and distinguish. Moreover, in elderly patients, clinical manifestation is minimal with abdominal discomfort, constipation, or fatigue, symptoms that most people tend to ignore as minor or non-perilous (**Figure 2**) [14, 15].

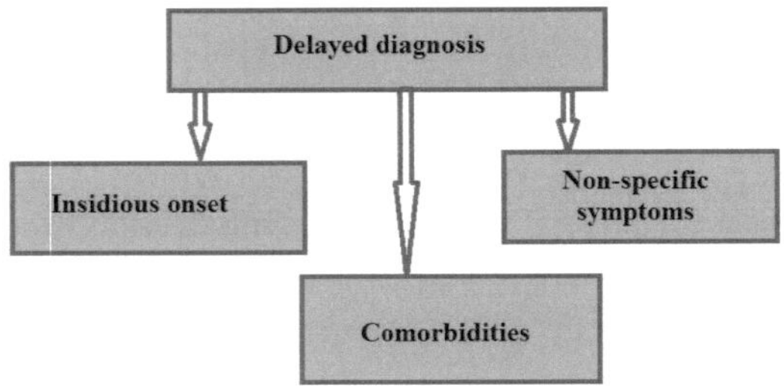

Figure 2. Factors associated with delayed diagnosis.

4. Diagnosis

Due to the fact that the nature of this disease is insidious, the diagnosis represents a challenge for clinicians. With the ever-increasing demographic shifts, more cases are now detected in areas where TB was a rarity until present. Unless a high degree of suspicion is maintained, the diagnosis can easily be missed or delayed [12].

Diagnostic techniques and procedures include:

- Clinical observation
- Imaging techniques: ultrasound, CT/MRI
- Laboratory tests
- Ascites fluid microbiologic and biochemical analysis

Generally, diagnosis is based on clinical suspicion, imaging of tuberculous infected zone, and detection of *M. tuberculosis* in ascitic fluid using acid-fast bacillus staining or culturing. The sensitivity of standard diagnostic methods such as Ziehl-Neelsen staining of smears and Lowenstein-Jensen culture done from ascitic fluid is very low for the diagnosis of abdominal TB. Ziehl-Neelsen staining of the ascitic fluid for mycobacterial detection is positive in only about 3% of the cases with proven TB peritonitis. Detection of mycobacteria requires the presence of more than 5000 bacilli/mL of specimen. In comparison, for positive culture, the presence of at least 10 organisms is considered to be sufficient. For a successful detection, culture methods based on a combination of liquid or biphasic media, together with solid media, are necessary [16, 17].

Nucleic acid amplification tests (NAATs) are molecular diagnostic methods based on amplification of mycobacterial nucleic acid. These are rapid methods that provide results within a day, and they are more specific and sensitive than Acid-Fast Bacillus Smear (AFB) smear. Albeit NAATs were originally designed for respiratory specimens, they can also be used on specimens from other TB sites like ascitic fluid samples, but this technique is still under evaluation.

Ascites of TB peritonitis obtained through ultrasound-guided paracentesis is an exudative type, and macroscopically its appearance is chylous and cloudy or turbid. Biochemically, the serum-ascites albumin gradient (SAAG) is now considered a more sensitive and specific measure than the ascitic total protein concentration which has been used for many years, in differentiating the ascites due to portal hypertension from ascites due to other pathophysiological mechanisms, such as tuberculous ascites which has a SAAG <1.1 g/dL and total proteins $>3–4$ g% [18, 19]. Combining LDH with total protein analysis has been explored for ascitic fluid. The cutoff values for three parameters in the ascitic fluid for differentiation between hepatic and non-hepatic ascites are as follows: LDH of 400 Sigma units, fluid/serum total protein (TP) ratio of 0.5, and fluid/serum LDH ratio of 0.6. The presence of any two of these three findings is usually associated with TB; the absence of all three indicates a hepatic cause [20].

Glucose concentration in the ascitic fluid, under normal conditions, is similar to that in the serum. Ascitic glucose concentration decreases due to consumption by bacteria, white blood cells, or cancer cells in the fluid in TB peritonitis. Ascitic glucose concentration is lower than normal in TB ascites, which makes it an indicator in differentiating tuberculosis from other diseases, such as cirrhosis. The ascitic/blood glucose ratio is a useful test in differentiating TB peritonitis from other causes of ascites [18].

Ascitic fluid adenosine deaminase activity (ADA) is considered a more sensitive and specific method used for early diagnosis of TB ascites. Even if the full physiological role of ADA is not yet completely understood, it is known that ADA values are notably higher (>40 U/L) in patients with TB ascites [21–23].

Non-biochemical tests of ascitic fluid, including cell counts, bacterial culture, and polymerase chain reaction (PCR), have an important role in diagnosing the cause of ascites.

The total cell count in tuberculous ascites is 150–4000/μL, and the cytologic examination shows over 70–80% lymphocytes and more than 250 leucocytes/mm^3 (**Table 1**).

The sensitivity of direct microscopic smear detection of acid-fast bacilli in the ascitic fluid (0–6%) and ascitic fluid mycobacterial culture (20–35%) is low, and because of the delay in obtaining the results of mycobacterial cultures of ascitic fluid, the mortality is high, and the value of these tests in the differential diagnosis of ascites is limited.

Recently, a new approach to the fast diagnosis of bacterial infections emerged, including tuberculosis. The advanced molecular techniques provided a new method represented by PCR which can detect minimal amounts of bacterial DNA and improves the rates of bacterial identification from 4 to 6 weeks for microbiological cultures to 24 hours. In diagnosing TB effusions, PCR appears to be an ideal tool, with 94% sensitivity and 88% specificity, becoming a rapid and reliable method for identification of infectious ascites [24].

The tuberculin skin testing (TST or purified protein derivative (PPD) skin test) is controversial, despite the high specificity of this test which is between 95 and 99%. Skin testing is currently used only for detection of latent infection because of its low sensitivity and low positive predictive value. At the moment, there are no recommendations for using this test to diagnose active

Type	Exudative
Appearance	Chylous and cloudy/turbid
Total cell count	150–4000/μL
Leucocytes	>250/mm^3
Lymphocytes	>70–80%
Total proteins	>3–4 g%
ADA	>40 U/L
LDH	>400 SU
Glucose	<6 mg/dL
SAAG	<1.1 g/dL

Table 1. Characteristics of tuberculous ascites.

disease like tuberculous peritonitis. At best, tuberculin skin testing can only offer auxiliary information. Several studies have reported positivity rates ranging between 24 and 100% with no significant difference between high and low endemicity areas. Currently, the recommendations about the cut point for the induration differ depending on the risk scale. For patients at low risk, the cut point is at 15 mm; in cases of moderate risk, the cut point is 10 mm, and for those at high risk, the cut point is 5 mm. Generally, about 50% of the patients would have false-negative reactions to this test, suggesting the fact that it has many potential sources of error. In conclusion, anergy testing may yield confusing information and is no longer recommended for diagnosis [25].

A great scientific advance has been the development of an IFN-c-based test with an 89% sensitivity, which is a quantitative in vitro assay evaluating the cell-mediated immune response to *M. tuberculosis* and has excellent agreement with tuberculin skin testing. The principle of this test is that previously sensitized T lymphocytes release IFN-c in response to stimulation by purified protein derivative (PPD).

In the past few years, the tuberculin skin test has been replaced by T-cell-based interferon-gamma release assay (IGRA) which is more sensitive and more specific. IGRA is an in vitro test used in all circumstances in which the TST is currently used, including evaluation of immigrants, surveillance programs, or contact investigations [26]. There are three commercially available IFN-γ tests: QuantiFERON-TB Gold assay (QFN-Gold), QuantiFERON-TB Gold *In-Tube* assay (QFN-G-IT), and T-SPOT.TB assay. They are rapid immunodiagnostic tests that can detect interferon-γ (IFN-γ) produced by lymphocytes in response to *Mycobacterium tuberculosis* (MTB). T-SPOT.TB test is a blood IFN-γ assay that measures the number of IFN-γ-producing T cells by identifying IFN-γ release when stimulated by MTB-specific antigens, including early secretory antigenic target 6 and culture filtrate protein 10, using enzyme-linked immunospot assay. QuantiFERON-TB Gold test is the predecessor of QuantiFERON-TB Gold In-Tube test, and they both measure production of IFN-γ in culture supernatant using enzyme-linked immunosorbent assay (ELISA). This measurement is possible by circulating T cells in whole blood being challenged with *M. tuberculosis*-specific antigens. The advantage of blood IGRA tests over tuberculin skin tests is the fact that IGRAs do not cross-react with the Bacillus of Calmette and Guérin (BCG) vaccine antigens, but suboptimal results can be possible in diagnosing EPTB because they aren't able to distinguish latent infection from active disease [27]. According to some researches, *M. tuberculosis* antigen-specific T cells may accumulate at infection sites; therefore, investigating body fluid IGRAs may increase the accuracy of EPTB diagnosis [28, 29].

Imaging techniques used for detection of TB ascites are ultrasound and computed tomography. These methods also increase the accuracy of several procedures like paracentesis or peritoneal biopsies, providing a safer and affordable replacement to diagnostic laparoscopy [30].

Ultrasound is the most sensitive and reliable method of detecting ascites, guiding paracentesis and monitoring the effects of therapy. It can detect even small volumes of fluid (as little as 100 ml of fluid could be detected). Ascites is usually seen as an anechoic space. In TB ascites, particulate matter within the ascitic fluid or fine, mobile strands, representing echogenic debris, can be detected. Less commonly, the ultrasound can reveal calcifications in the walls of encysted ascitic fluid [12].

On computed tomography the ascitic fluid has high attenuation values, between 20 and 45 HU, and the peritoneum is symmetrically thickened and nodular. Frequently, an early sign of abdominal TB is a thickened mesentery (>15 mm) with mesenteric lymph nodes.

Many studies concluded that ultrasonography and computed tomography are complementary to each other in detecting TB ascites, as they provide different details. CT focuses on the peritoneum and omental and mesentery involvement, and the ultrasound shows fine, mobile septations (**Figure 3**) [31].

However, the only certain way to diagnose TB ascites is the histological examination. Various methods that include excision, laparoscopy, needle biopsy and ultrasound-guided biopsies, endoscopy, computed tomography (CT), or endoscopic ultrasound are used to establish the

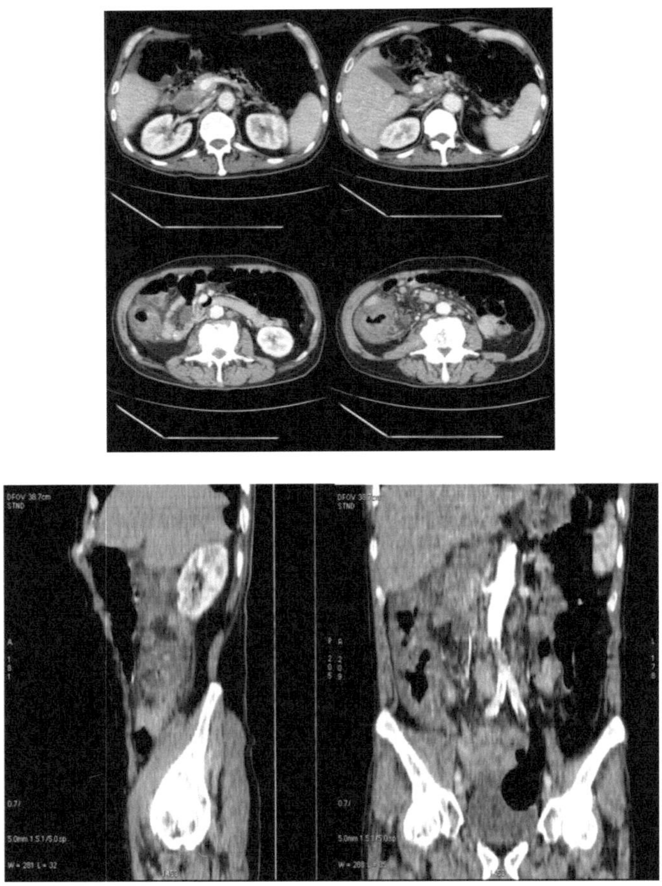

Figure 3. Circumferential parietal thickness, with an edematous appearance of the appendix, cecum, ascending colon, and up to the hepatic flexura, associating stripe thickening of adjacent fat. Multiple adenopathies containing calcifications and central necrosis. Fluid accumulation in the peritoneal cavity associating symmetrical, iodophilic thickening of parietal peritoneum. Osteolytic areas with an adjacent osteosclerotic reaction in L2, L3, and L4 vertebrae. Parafluid accumulation in L2–L3 and L3–L4 intervertebral spaces that reaches the anterior epidural space and the roots of L2 and L3 nerves, extending to L3–L4 adjacent smooth tissues, with no visible border toward the right psoas muscle.

diagnosis. The presence of granulomas is typical for TB ascites [32]. The relative sensitivities of different procedures and the potential therapeutic benefits should be considered in making the choice of diagnostic approach. In superficial TB lymphadenitis, fine needle aspiration (FNA) biopsy of affected lymph nodes is the gold-standard diagnostic technique. Excision biopsy has the highest sensitivity, whereas FNA is less invasive and may be useful. If FNA examination results are doubtful, excision biopsy may be needed. Laparoscopy with target peritoneal biopsy is the current first-line investigation in the diagnosis of peritoneal TB [33, 34]. Several studies revealed a diagnostic accuracy of 84–96% for TB peritonitis.

Generally, tissue biopsy is superior to fluid aspiration in providing positive culture results. The diagnosis is more accurate when the biopsy results and polymerase chain reaction assays are combined with culture results [35].

5. Differential diagnosis

The main differential diagnosis is peritoneal carcinomatosis, which can be difficult to distinguish, especially in older patients. The nodules of carcinomatosis are larger, usually more than 3 mm, more vascular, and more irregular than the tuberculous ones which rarely surpass 1–2 mm. Carcinomatosis is seen as an irregular peritoneal thickening with nodular implants, while TB peritonitis is suggested by the presence of a smooth peritoneum with symmetrical thickening, ascites, and enlarged lymph nodes of low attenuation [31].

Other less likely considerations include:

- Ascites in liver diseases: the liver is enlarged and irregular; proteins are lower than 4 g%.
- Nephrotic syndrome: ascites is less marked; proteins are lower than 4 g%.
- Nutritional edema (hypoproteinemia) has many other signs of protein deficiency; proteins are also lower than 4 g%.
- Starch peritonitis, sarcoidosis, and Crohn's disease may resemble the laparoscopic features of TB peritonitis, but the presence of caseating granuloma establishes the diagnosis (**Table 2**) [36, 37].

The most important differential diagnosis	Less likely considerations
	Ascites in liver disease
	Nephrotic syndrome
Peritoneal carcinomatosis	Hypoproteinemia
	Sarcoidosis
	Starch peritonitis
	Crohn's disease

Table 2. Differential diagnosis.

There are a few signs that additionally suggest the diagnosis of TB peritonitis: normal serum levels of CA 19–9 and carcinoembryonic antigen (CEA), elevated serum levels of CA 125, fever, and lymphocyte-predominant benign ascites, but only biopsies yield the final diagnosis [38, 39].

6. Treatment

Treatment is initiated not only in patients with confirmed diagnosis but also in patients with strong suspicion of TB, because a delay in treatment initiation can lead to significant mortality. TB treatment initiation includes also individuals with ascites associated with fever, weight loss, imaging signs of TB, personal history of TB, or contact with a tuberculosis case.

Despite the fact that most guidelines on the treatment of tuberculosis suggest that 6 months of treatment is sufficient for extrapulmonary tuberculosis (except for the case of bone tuberculosis or tuberculous meningitis), most physicians treating peritoneal tuberculosis use antituberculous therapy for 9 to 12 months [40, 41].

Drug treatment is the most important modality and follows standard regimens and principles. There are currently five drugs that are considered first-line medications: isoniazid, rifampicin, pyrazinamide, streptomycin, and ethambutol. Second-line drugs are only used in case of resistance to first-line therapy (extensively drug-resistant tuberculosis or multidrug-resistant tuberculosis), and they are represented by aminoglycosides, fluoroquinolones, polypeptides, cycloserine, thioamides, and terizidone. There is also a third-line therapy with uncertain or unproven efficacy including rifabutin, macrolides, linezolid, thioacetazone, thioridazine, arginine, bedaquiline, and vitamin D [42]. Drug-resistant disease varies substantially in different areas of the world and may occur in cases of poor patient management, nonadherence to prescribed regimen, or as a result of malabsorption of the antituberculous drugs.

The treatment of TB peritonitis in patients with HIV is usually the same, but because HIV-infected patients are often taking multiple drugs, some of which may interact with antituberculous ones; it is strongly recommended to consult the experts in HIV-related TB.

The "complete response" to antituberculous treatment means complete resolution of symptoms and ascites within 6 months; in most cases, laboratory tests return to normal values within 3 months. Persistence of ascites means "no response" [43, 44].

7. Conclusions

Peritoneal tuberculosis is still common in areas of the world where TB is prevalent and its incidence ratio is likely to increase as a consequence of population migrations.

Ascites can be a complication of an aggregate of diseases, which carries an unfavorable prognosis that depends on the causes, the moment of diagnosis, and the start of the treatment.

Establishing the diagnosis of TB ascites requires a high index of suspicion because of its insidious development. In any patient with several weeks of abdominal pain, weight loss, fever, and lymphocytic dominant ascites with SAAG < 1.1 g/L, as well as in patients with ascites belonging to special population groups, such as indigenous or older people, or patients with ascites as the primary symptom, ascitic TB peritonitis should be considered in differential diagnosis. This syndrome behaves clinically like many abdominal diseases that are often ignored, leading to a significant impact on morbidity and mortality due to a delayed diagnosis and treatment. Older laboratory tests lack sensitivity and specificity in establishing the diagnosis. Histological examination, considered the gold-standard diagnosis method, is an invasive procedure with high risk of complications. More accurate methods such as molecular tests based on mycobacterial nucleic acid amplification tests (NAATs), PCR techniques used to detect bacterial DNA, or interferon-gamma release assays (IGRA) and biochemical methods such as the serum-ascites albumin gradient (SAAG), ratio between LDH in ascites fluid/serum total protein (TP) ratio and fluid ascites/serum LDH ratio, adenosine deaminase activity (ADA), and imagistic techniques were recently considered for an efficient positive diagnosis of TB ascites, making possible the early treatment with appropriate tuberculostatic drugs.

Author details

Andra-Iulia Suceveanu*, Despina Todescu, Laura Mazilu, Filippos Goniotakis Manousos, Roxana Hulea, Felix Voinea, Eugen Dumitru and Adrian Paul Suceveanu

*Address all correspondence to: andrasuceveanu@yahoo.com

Faculty of Medicine, Ovidius University, Constanta, Romania

References

[1] Dye C, Lönnroth K, Jaramillo E, et al. Trends in tuberculosis incidence and their determinants in 134 countries. Bulletin of the World Health Organization. 2009;87:683

[2] Walter ND, Jasmer RM, Grinsdale J, et al. Reaching the limits of tuberculosis prevention among foreign-born individuals: A tuberculosis-control program perspective. Clinical Infectious Diseases. 2008;46:103. DOI: 10.1086/523733

[3] Canadian Thoracic Society and The Public Health Agency of Canada and Licensors. Canadian Tuberculosis Standards. 7th ed. Ottawa: Public Health Agency of Canada; 2013. pp. 247-273

[4] Schluger NW, Rom WN. The host immune response to tuberculosis. American Journal of Respiratory and Critical Care Medicine. 1998;157:679-691

[5] Mehta JB, Dutt A, Harvill L, Mathews KM. Epidemiology of extrapulmonary tuberculosis. A comparative analysis with pre-AIDS era. Chest. 1991;99:1134

[6] Gherasim L. Non-surgical diseases of the peritoneum - Ascites. Internal Medicine. Vol. 3. Ed. Medicala; 1998. pp. 1159-1176

[7] Lazarus A, Thilagar B. Abdominal Tuberculosis. Disease-a-Month. 2007;53(1):32-38

[8] Dineen P, Homan WP, Grafe WR. Tuberculous peritonitis: 43 years experience in diagnosis and treatment. Annals of Surgery. 1976;184:717-722

[9] Sanai FM, Bzeizi KI. Systematic review: Tuberculous peritonitis—presenting features, diagnostic strategies and treatment. Alimentary Pharmacology and Therapeutics. 2005;22(8): 685-700

[10] Lin-Lin H, Harry Hua-Xiang X, Sen-Lin Z. Ascitic Fluid Analysis in the Differential Diagnosis of Ascites: Focus on Cirrhotic Ascites. Available from: https://www.ncbi.nlm.nih.gov/pmc/articles/PMC4521252

[11] Chow KM, Chow VC, Hung LC, Wong SM, Szeto CC. Tuberculous peritonitis-associated mortality is high among patients waiting for the results of mycobacterial cultures of ascitic fluid samples. Clinical Infectious Diseases. 2002;35:409-413

[12] Jain R, Sawhney S, Bhargava DK, Berry M. Diagnosis of abdominal tuberculosis: Sonographic findings in patients with early disease. American Journal of Roentgenology. 1995;165:1391-1395

[13] Bernhard JS, Bhatia G, Knauer CM. Gastrointestinal tuberculosis: An eighteen-patient experience and review. Journal of Clinical Gastroenterology. 2000;30:397-402

[14] Al Karawi MA, Mohamed AE, Yasawy MI, et al. Protean manifestations of gastrointestinal tuberculosis: Report on 130 patients. Journal of Clinical Gastroenterology. 1995;20: 225-232

[15] Gonnella JS, Hudson EK. Clinical patterns of tuberculous peritonitis. Archives of Internal Medicine. 1966;117:164-169

[16] Yeager HJ Jr, Lacy J, Smith L, LeMaistre C. Quantitative studies of mycobacterial populations in sputum and saliva. The American Review of Respiratory Disease. 1967;95: 998-1004

[17] Gupta S, Kumari S, Banwalikar JN, Gupta SK. Diagnostic utility of the estimation of mycobacterial antigen A60 specific immunoglobulins IgM, IgA and IgG in the sera of cases of adult human tuberculosis. Tubercle and Lung Disease. 1995;76:418-424

[18] Tarn AC, Lapworth R. Biochemical analysis of ascitic (peritoneal) fluid: What should we measure? Annals of Clinical Biochemistry. 2010;47:397-407

[19] Mansour-Ghanaei F, Shafaghi A, Bagherzadeh AH, Fallah MS. Low gradient ascites: A seven year course review. World Journal of Gastroenterology. 2005;11:2337-2339

[20] Sevinc A, Sari R, Fadillioglu E. The utility of lactate dehydrogenase isoenzyme pattern in the diagnostic evaluation of malignant and nonmalignant ascites. Journal of the National Medical Association. 2005;97:79-84

[21] Riquelme A, Calvo M, Salech F, et al. Value of adenosine deaminase (ADA) in ascitic fluid for the diagnosis of tuberculous peritonitis: A meta-analysis. Journal of Clinical Gastroenterology. 2006;40(8):705-710

[22] Segura RM, Pascual C, Ocana I, et al. Adenosine deaminase in body fluids: A useful diagnostic tool in tuberculosis. Clinical Biochemistry. 1989;22:141-148

[23] Blake J, Berman P. The use of adenosine deaminase assays in the diagnosis of tuberculosis. South African Medical Journal. 1982;62:19-23

[24] Schwake L, von Herbay A, Junghanss T, Stremmel W, Mueller M. Peritoneal tuberculosis with negative polymerase chain reaction results: Report of two cases. Scandinavian Journal of Gastroenterology. 2003;38:221-224

[25] Arend SM, van Meijgaarden KE, de Boer K, de Palou EC, van Soolingen D, Ottenhoff TH, van Dissel JT. Tuberculin skin testing and in vitro T cell responses to ESAT-6 and culture filtrate protein 10 after infection with *Mycobacterium marinum* or *M. kansasii*. The Journal of Infectious Diseases. 2002;186:1797-1807

[26] Pai M, Zwerling A, Menzies D. Systematic review: T cell-based assays for the diagnosis of latent tuberculosis infection: An update. Annals of Internal Medicine. 2008;149:177-184

[27] Wagner D, Hörster R, Lange B, Lange C. Evaluation of T-cell interferon-gamma-release assays for the diagnosis of latent and active tuberculosis. Deutsche Medizinische Wochenschrift. 2008;133:354-357

[28] Sharma SK, Tahir M, Mohan A, Smith-Rohrberg D, Mishra HK, Pandey RM. Diagnostic accuracy of ascitic fluid IFN-gamma and adenosine deaminase assays in the diagnosis of tuberculous ascites. Journal of Interferon & Cytokine Research. 2006;26:484-488

[29] Greco S, Girardi E, Masciangelo R, Capoccetta GB, Saltini C. Adenosine deaminase and interferon measurements for the diagnosis of tuberculous pleurisy: A meta-analysis. The International Journal of Tuberculosis and Lung Disease. 2003;7:777-786

[30] Burrill J, Williams CJ, Bain G, et al. Tuberculosis: A radiologic review. Radiographics. 2007;27(5):1255-1273

[31] Ha HK, Jung JI, Lee MS, et al. CT differentiation of tuberculous peritonitis and peritoneal carcinomatosis. AJR American Journal of Roentgenology. 1996;167:743-748

[32] Mimica M. The usefulness and limitations of laparoscopy in the diagnosis of tuberculous peritonitis. Endoscopy. 1992;24:588-591

[33] Barry RE, Brown P, Read AE. Physicians use of laparoscopy. British Medical Journal. 1978;2:1276-1278

[34] Chu CM, Lin SM, Peng SM, et al. The role of laparoscopy in the evaluation of ascites of unknown origin. Gastrointestinal Endoscopy. 1994;40:285-289

[35] Bhargava DK, Shriniwas, Chopra P, et al. Peritoneal tuberculosis: Laparoscopic patterns and its diagnostic accuracy. The American Journal of Gastroenterology. 1992;87:109-112

[36] McHutchison JG. Differential diagnosis of ascites. Seminars in Liver Disease. 1997;17:191-202

[37] Alexandrakis MG, Moschandrea JA, Koulocheri SA, Kouroumalis E, Eliopoulos GD. Discrimination between malignant and nonmalignant ascites using serum and ascitic fluid proteins in a multivariate analysis model. Digestive Diseases and Sciences. 2000;45:500-508

[38] Louhimo J, Finne P, Alfthan H, Stenman UH, Haglund C. Combination of HCG beta, CA 19-9, and CEA with logistic regression improves accuracy in gastrointestinal malignancies. Anticancer Research. 2002;22:1759-1764

[39] Xiao W, Liu Y. Elevation of serum and ascites cancer antigen 125 levels in patients with liver cirrhosis. Journal of Gastroenterology and Hepatology. 2003;18:1315-1316

[40] Treatment Duration for Abdominal Tuberculosis. July, 2015. Available from: https://clinicaltrials.gov/ct2/show/NCT01124929 [Accessed 2 March 2016]

[41] World Health Organization. Guidelines on the Management of Latent Tuberculosis Infection. Geneva: WHO; 2015. Available from: http://www.who.int/tb/publications/ltbi_document_page/en/[Accessed 2 March 2016]

[42] Lonnroth K, Castro KG, Chakaya JM, Chauhan LS, Floyd K, Glaziou P, Raviglione MC. Tuberculosis control and elimination 2010-50: Cure, care, and social development. Lancet. 2010;375:1814-1829

[43] Lonnroth K, Uplekar M. Invest in breaking the barriers of public-private collaboration for improved tuberculosis care. Bulletin of the World Health Organization. 2005;83:558-559

[44] Mendez A, Raviglione MC, Laszlo A, Binkin N, Rieder HL, Bustreo F,Cohn DL, Lambregts-vanWeezenbeek CS, Kim SJ, Chaulet P, et al. Global surveillance for antituberculosis-drug resistance, 1994-1997. World Health Organization-International Union against Tuberculosis and Lung Disease Working Group on Anti-Tuberculosis Drug Resistance Surveillance. The New England Journal of Medicine. 1998;338:1641-1649

Chapter 4

Ascitic Fluid in Ovarian Carcinoma – From Pathophysiology to the Treatment

Radomir Živadinović, Aleksandra Petrić, Dane Krtinić, Sonja Pop-Trajković Dinić and Biljana Živadinović

Additional information is available at the end of the chapter

http://dx.doi.org/10.5772/intechopen.70476

Abstract

Due to low symptomatology, a lack of screening, and relatively complicated diagnostic procedures of ovarian carcinoma, more and more women are believed to visit their doctors in advanced stage of the disease, complicated with ascitic fluid. There is an increasing evidence that peritoneal cytology is a subjective assessment with certain percentage of false-positive and false-negative results that may cause application of unnecessary chemotherapy or nonapplication of necessary chemotherapy. Maximal cytoreductive surgery followed by intraperitoneal or systemic chemotherapy remains to be the gold standard in preventing ascites. Ascites is not only a symptom of a disease, but a specific microenvironment for formation and mediation of protumorigenic signals that control ovarian cancer progression, proliferation, invasion, anti-apoptosis, chemoresistance and tumor heterogeneity. Acellular cytokines and immunological factors influence ovarian cancer progression and its ability to prevent immune responses of the body and tumor reaction to chemotherapy. Ascites contributes to disease dissemination, changing its course and final outcomes. Management of patients with ascites and ovarian carcinoma is complex and often the goal of the treatment is to target palliative procedures. Multidisciplinary approach is necessary in the management of these patients. Further investigations of new drugs and immunomodulators are needed aiming at prolonged periods between relapses.

Keywords: ovarian carcinoma, ascitic fluid, treatment, cytological findings, immunohistochemical markers

1. Introduction

Ascitic fluid is the presence of large volumes of fluid accumulated in the abdominal cavity. Normally, several liters of peritoneal fluid are produced and it is not accumulated, but effectively absorbed. This fluid continuously circulates in a clockwise direction helping in the lubrication of intestines.

Malignant ascites accounts for about 10% of all cases of ascites [1]. Causes of nonmalignant ascites are: liver diseases (cirrhosis), congestive heart failure, and occlusion of the inferior vena cava or the hepatic vein occlusion, as well as benign tumors of the genital tract (ovarian fibromas). Malignant ascites are most commonly found with gynecological neoplasms (primarily ovarian and endometrial cancer), gastrointestinal malignancies, and breast cancer. In 15–30% of cases, the ascites is associated with carcinomatosis of the endometrium [2].

According to traditional classification, ascites is divided into exudative and transudative types. Ninety percent of ascitic fluids are transudates resulting from nonmalignant conditions, such as congestive heart failure or liver cirrhosis. Physical characteristics include clear appearance of the fluid with the presence of few cells (acellular) and low albumin level. On the other hand, exudates are most commonly malignant (ovarian carcinoma), with usually cloudy appearance of fluid, increased cellular count, and higher albumin level in comparison to transudates [3].

A new term used to assist in determining such a classification is the serum-ascites albumin gradient (SAAG).

This gradient is defined like the difference between albumin concentration of serum and ascitic fluid. If the gradient is >1.1, it indicates transudates due to portal hypertension, cirrhosis, hepatic congestion, portal vein thrombosis, etc. If SAAG <1.1, it indicates exudates not related to portal hypertension, but mostly malignant etiology (ovarian carcinoma), peritoneal carcinomatosis, chronic peritoneal infection, nephrotic syndrome, or hypoalbuminemia [4].

Besides protein concentrations, ascitic fluid may additionally be analyzed by macroscopic and microscopic testing.

Macroscopic testing means the analysis of appearance and color of ascites. Cloudy physical characteristics indicate the presence of leukocytes, infection, or malignancy. Yellow color is more common in liver diseases, greenish results from the bile, and reddish color may indicate the presence of hemorrhage.

Chemical tests, in addition to albumin concentration, include glucose level concentration (lower with infection), amylase (increased with pancreatitis), and lactate dehydrogenase (increased in carcinomas). If an infection is suspected, Gram stain analyses may be performed, as well as bacterial culture testing, viral testing, and microbacterial testing (tuberculosis).

Microscopic examination is performed if infectious or malignant ascites is suspected. Total cell count or leukocyte counting and differentiation are performed to determine infectious etiology more precisely. If malignant etiology is suspected, the most important thing is to determine the presence or absence of the cells with atypical morphological characteristics or malignant cells.

2. Pathophysiology

The pathophysiology of malignant ascites is multifactorial and is related to a combination of two basic pathogenic mechanism, increased vascular permeability and obstructed lymphatic drainage.

Five microscopic barriers prevent movement of proteins away from vascular space: capillary endothelium, capillary basement membrane, interstitial stroma, mesothelial basement membrane, and mesothelial cells. In 1922, Putnam described the peritoneal membrane as a living, dynamic membrane through which the electrolytes pass between the peritoneum and serum. The movement of colloid solutions from serum is not clear enough and presents the relative impermeability through intercellular spaces based on Starling's law of osmotic gradient. The exchange of fluid between the plasma and interstitium is based on the hydraulic and osmotic pressure. Oncotic pressure is based on fluid reabsorption from the interstitial space and edema prevention. Macromolecules, proteins and cells that accumulate in the peritoneal cavity may return to the systemic circulation by means of peritoneal lymphatic system and lymphatic stomata to lymphatics that lead to the diaphragm and the thoracic duct [5].

In 1953, Holm and Nielson demonstrated the importance of lymphatic obstruction in pathogenesis of malignant ascites. The basic characteristics of malignant ascites include increased ascitic fluid protein concentration, increase of lactate dehydrogenase, large number of leukocytes, and positive cytology regarding the presence of malignant cells. High protein concentration in the peritoneal cavity results from vascular permeability due to increased vascular endothelial growth factor (VEGF) levels. The concentration of VEGF is significantly higher in malignant ascites than in nonmalignant ascites (cirrhosis). Splanchnic hyperemia and tumor necrosis factor dominate in nonmalignant ascites.

The complete pathogenic mechanism of malignant ascites is still not well understood. The events that are definitely happening and that we are familiar with include an increase of net filtration and accumulation of ascitic fluid resulting from increased capillary permeability, increased surface area for filtration, increased hydraulic pressure difference, and decreased oncotic pressure difference [6].

A two-way permeability of blood vessels is necessary for tissue normal supply with nutrients, gases, minor proteins, and waste removal. It can be basal, acute vascular (a consequence of short exposure to VEGF) and chronic, characteristic of pathological (malignant) angiogenesis.

Apart from the most important aforementioned VEGF that stimulates vascular permeability, other factors responsible for stimulation include basic fibroblast growth factor (bFGF), angiogenin, transforming growth factors (TGF α and β), and interleukin-8. All these factors lead to neovascularization and angiogenesis, starting with endothelium stimulation and resulting in hyperpermeability and degradation of endothelial membrane, followed by migration and proliferation of endothelial cells and the development of new capillaries. VEGF has been identified in ovary tumor cells, with its overexpression reported in ovarian carcinoma.

Neoangiogenesis and an increase of peritoneal blood vessels in size and number result not only in increased permeability but also in increased overall surface area for filtration. The next pathogenic mechanism of malignant ascites is increased hydrostatic pressure difference as a result of minor elevation of portal venous pressure in patients with ovarian cancer (portal veins compression by tumor mass and metastases). On the other hand, the oncotic pressure difference is reduced since the albumins that are responsible for osmotic intravascular pressure (reabsorbs fluid from the interstitial space) degrade into smaller peptides or amino acids (increased production of metalloproteinase).

Of all of these pathogenic mechanisms, it can be concluded that the main cause of ascites is not tumor, but peritoneal surface by indirect action of cytokine mediators (VEGF, etc.).

3. Clinical manifestation and ascites as a prognostic factor

Ascites is the most common symptom in patients with ovarian carcinoma and the reason for visiting a doctor. In 54% of patients with peritoneal carcinomatosis, ascites was the first detectable sign of malignancy [7].

Unfortunately, the presence of ascites most commonly reveals an advanced stage of the disease, since ascites are produced in only 7% in I and II stages of the disease and in 89% in stages III and IV. The amount of ascetic fluid is in correlation with the stage of the disease, for stages I and II its presence is < 0.5 L, but in more than 66% of cases with stages III and IV its presence is > 0.5 L.

More than 2/3 of patients report to their doctors in stages III and IV that when ascites increased abdominal size and abdominal distension, dyspnea, weight gain, lower extremity edema, nausea and vomiting, the phenomenon of fluid wave, and shifting dullness occur. Survival rate in advanced stages of the disease (III and IV) is 5–20% [8].

The presence of ascitic fluid less than 100 ml is without symptoms and impossible to detect gynecologically. In 14% of cases, such as small amounts of ascites are not detected by ultrasound examination either. However, ultrasonography is important not only in detecting ascites but also in its quantification and localization in paracentesis.

CT scans have an important role in detection and are potent in showing peritoneal carcinomatosis, omental involvement, and peritoneal ischemia. Paracentesis, laparoscopy, and laparotomy assist in final determination of the amount, biochemical, and cytological origin of ascitic fluid, as well as primary localization of tumor that caused the production of ascitic fluid (immunohistochemistry and markers).

Ascites is a grave prognostic marker. The presence of malignant ascites in malignomas of other location (pancreas, stomach, large intestine, breasts) is a poor prognostic parameter, with survival rate of 7–13 weeks from the time of detection. In ovarian carcinoma, survival rate is longest, more than 19 weeks. Unfavorable prognostic parameter is depressed serum albumin, as well as depressed serum ascites albumin (transudate) [9].

4. Cytology, biochemistry, and immunohistochemistry of ascitic fluid

The first report on peritoneal fluid cytology aimed at detecting subclinical metastases was published in 1950. FIGO introduced peritoneal washing cytology in staging of ovarian carcinoma in 1973. Positive cytological finding is important for substaging of I and II stages of the disease (I and II c stages) and is an important predictive prognostic and recurrence factor. However, more and more studies show that morphologic examination of cytological samples, associated with therapeutic and prognostic implications, is not a diagnostic tool with high sensitivity. Malignant cells may be few in number and hardly recognized among numerous mesothelial cells and macrophages. On the other hand, mesothelial cells exhibiting reactive changes (with enlarged hyperchromatic nuclei and cytoplasmic alterations) may be misinterpreted as neoplastic cells, thus resulting in stage upgrading and unnecessary chemotherapy.

Reactive mesothelial cells - enlarged, with dense cytoplasm, enlarged nucleus with nucleolus, may be vacuolated, or contain cellular windows. Endosalpingiosis displays organized clusters with uniform and scant basophilic cytoplasm cells, the nucleus with normal membrane, a fine chromatin, and small nucleoli. Endometriosis, as another diagnostic error, shows the presence of round cells arranged in three-dimensional clusters and layers, round and bean-shaped nucleus with fine chromatin, and scant and vacuolated cytoplasm. The most sensitive finding in endometriosis is the presence of macrophages with hemosiderin.

For all of these reasons, peritoneal cytology may be false positive in even 4.5% of cases. On the other hand, the false-negative rate is high and accounts for more than 20%. The factors that are responsible for such a false-negative rate may include poor distribution of washings, infrequent exfoliation of cells, and interpretive errors [10].

Cytological manifestation of serous carcinoma presents single cells or poorly cohesive irregular cell clusters, with large pleomorphic nucleus and prominent nucleolus. Cytological manifestation of endometrioid carcinoma shows three-dimensional cluster of cells with large eccentric and pleomorphic nucleus, coarse chromatin, prominent nucleolus, and abundant cytoplasm.

One of our study showed reliability and limitations of cytological analysis of ascites in ovarian carcinoma. The experimental group was composed of 76 cytological findings obtained from patients diagnosed with ovarian carcinoma, whereas the control group included 94 cytological findings of benign ovarian tumors and ascites in liver cirrhosis. **Table 1** shows distribution of false-negative cytological findings of ascitic fluid with respect to the histological type of tumor. **Table 2** shows distribution of false-positive peritoneal cytological findings with respect to the cause and histological type of tumor. In that study, it was concluded that peritoneal cytology of ascitic fluid is highly specific (93.61%) but it has a relatively low sensitivity (68.92%). In 30.02%, peritoneal cytology had false-negative results, and in 6.38%, it showed false-positive results [11].

The sensitivity of peritoneal cytology according to literature data is as low as 50–60% and as high as 97%, depending on the study, the stage of the disease, and the involvement of the peritoneum [12].

Histological type	Total number of histological type	Number of negative cytological findings	Percentage of false-negative findings
Serous	54	15	27.77
Mucinous	6	2	33.33
Endometrioid	4	3	77
Clear cell	6	2	33.33
Anaplastic	4	1	25
Granulocellular	2	0	0
Total	76	23	30.2

Table 1. Distribution of false-negative cytological findings of ascitic fluid with respect to the histological type of tumor.

In patients with stage Ic and ruptured capsule, cytology is positive in 75% and with peritoneal involvement in 94% cases [13]. Cytology sensitivity in peritoneal involvement is 82.9% and specificity 98.1% [14]. Some other authors found in their studies that the sensitivity of total validity of cytology to be somewhat lower than 60% with almost 100% specificity [15].

Upon the completion of the treatment, the results of secondary cytology are an important and independent prognostic marker that highly correlates with optimal effects of surgical treatment, recurrence, and overall survival rate. Thus, in positive secondary cytology, survival rate is 13–32 months, and in negative >48 months [16].

In order to improve total validity of peritoneal cytology, as well as cervical cytology, immunohistochemical and biochemical biomarkers are found to be useful. Among other things, the concentration of alkaline phosphatase level (in malignant ascites it is > 350 mg/dl), lactate dehydrogenase, fibronectin, telomerase, as well as tumor markers CA – 125, CEA, p53, and β-HCG plays an important role.

Histological type	Total number of histological type	Number of positive cytological findings	Percentage of false-positive findings
Fibroma	9	0	0
Dermoid	11	0	0
Endometrioma	13	2	15.38
Serous	39	2	5.12
Mucinous	20	2	10
Liver cirrhosis	2	0	0
Total	94	6	6.38

Table 2. Distribution of false-positive peritoneal cytology findings with respect to the cause and histological type of tumor.

http://dx.doi.org/10.5772/intechopen.70476

There is also a specific group of panel antibodies, primarily MOC-31 and Ber-EP4, highly effective in distinguishing mesothelial from cancerous cells. This differentiation may be supported by separation of antibodies into adherent cells (AD) (mesothelial and mesenchymal) and nonadherent (NAD) cells [17].

Telomerase has been the most tested biomarker lately. It is an enzyme essential for normal replication of chromosomes and constant growth of cancer cells (via telomere). In most somatic cells, telomerase activity is not expressed. On the other hand, in almost 100% of ovarian carcinoma, increased expression of telomerase activity has been proved. A special importance of the role of telomerase activity is in predicting the recurrence of the disease and in the post-treatment follow-up it is aimed at the detection of early recurrence. Contrary to 24–54% of cases with diagnosed residual disease, cytology, and second-look surgery negative, telomerase was found to be almost 100% positive [18]. The main limitation of this telomerase (TRAP) assay in wide clinical application is the rate of false-positive results in dermoid tumors and in some inflammatory processes.

Moreover, a recent study by Zhu et al. explored the values of tumor markers in serum and ascites for identifying and diagnosing malignant ascites by analyzing the clinical data of patients diagnosed with ascites; their findings suggested that compared to a single index, combined detection of tumor markers in the serum and ascites will significantly improve diagnostic sensitivity and specificity [19].

5. Ascites as a prognostic marker

Malignant ascites is a sign associated with malignant disease. The presence of ascitic fluid in ovarian cancer plays a major, even a key role in further progression of the malignant disease. The spread of ovarian cancer and the occurrence of peritoneal and abdominal metastases depend on ascitic fluid.

Specific cellular and acellular components of ascites provide tumor-friendly microenvironment, which not only promotes tumor cell growth and motility but also inhibits the positive response of chemotherapy, thus directly promoting chemoresistance in tumor cells [20, 21].

Available literature data on the disease progression and recurrence prove that metastases and recurrences may be prevented or reduced if the tumor is removed before being exposed to ascites and before tumor cells invade the peritoneum. Thus, for stage I disease, if the tumor is encapsulated and confined to the ovary, without ascites and without positive peritoneal washing, substage Ia, the recurrence rate accounts for 29%, but for the same stage I, substage Ic, with ascites and peritoneal washing positive for malignant cells, the recurrence rate expected is 59% [22].

Understanding the pathology of formation and reabsorption of ascites is necessary for demonstrating its impact on the disease progression and occurrence of metastases. Two thirds of the peritoneal fluid is reabsorbed by the lymphatic channels and reaches the diaphragm and the right subclavian vein by the negative intrathoracic pressure. Physiological factors that stimulate this flow are gravity, diaphragmatic pressure, organ mobility, and recesses formed by key anatomical structures [23]. There are three most common sites of ascites reabsorption and ovarian cancer metastasis, including the greater omentum, right subphrenic region, and pouch of Douglas, areas which have easy access to ascites [24].

On the other hand, the disease recurrence is almost always associated with the development of ascites. The most common and almost only therapeutic approach in the treatment of recurrences is chemotherapy. Chemoresistance and poor response to chemotherapy, often driven by the presence of ascites, directly correlate with survival rate and the disease recurrence. In chemoresistant tumors, a 5-year survival rate is less than 27% [25]. Thus, ascites indirectly affects a malignant disease prognosis, both by forming a specific microenvironment promoting tumor growth and by developing chemoresistance.

It is believed that future management options will focus more not only on surgical treatment of the disease but also on ascitic fluid and secondary malignant deposits treatment and chemoresistance as well, since the disease will already have spread beyond the ovaries in 75% of cases at the time of diagnosis [26].

6. Malignant ascites—immunological factors, cytokines, and acellular components

Common features of all malignant processes include hereditary and environmental factors and immunological factors as well. A balanced immune response, from immunopresentation to immune reaction or immune response, is an important factor of carcinogenesis. An immune response has to be timely, specific, and balanced. If early recognition of carcinogenic factors and genetic mutations fails and if Th1-, Th2-, and REG-mediated cellular immune response is hyporeactive or hyperreactive, then the progression of malignant processes occurs.

A study from 2017 based on a great number of papers from the Medline database showed that elevated neutrophil-to-lymphocyte ratio (NLR) could be an important diagnostic parameter predicative of poor prognosis for ovarian cancer. Elevation of NLR correlated with advanced FIGO stage (OR, 2.32; 95% CI, 1.79–3.00), higher serum level of CA-125 (OR, 3.33; 95% CI, 2.43–4.58), more extensive ascites (OR, 3.54; 95% CI, 2.31–5.42) as well as less chemotherapeutic response (OR, 0.53; 95% CI, 0.40–0.70) [27].

Inflammatory responses may be evaluated by the changes in leukocyte reaction, as well as by C-reactive protein (CRP) measurement. An elevated CPR level is also identified in cancer patients, and along with CA 125 tumor marker specific to ovarian cancer, it can be an excellent clinical and prognostic marker of a malignant disease [28].

An increase of inflammatory factors can be detected not only in the blood but also in tumor tissue and ascitic fluid. The concentration of cancer-associated soluble factors in ascites is much higher than in the serum. For all of these reasons, ascites is a specific and useful marker for investigating diagnostic, therapeutic, and prognostic factors regarding ovarian cancer.

Natural killer cells (NK) and T lymphocytes have significantly higher concentration in the ascites than in the blood in patients with ovarian cancer [29].

Cancer is a heterogeneous disease with cellular and molecular heterogeneity. Single nucleotide polymorphism (SNP) is also present. Apart from cellular heterogeneity, heterogeneity of ascitic fluid content, as well as measurements of inflammatory protein agent quantity, may be predictive of an aggressive tumor and serve as a useful prognostic marker. Besides inflammatory parameters, it is important to evaluate the presence or absence of oncogenic and tumor suppressive factors that have an impact on final outcome of the disease. Thus, ascites in high-grade serous ovarian cancer patients has been shown to serve as a protective tumor microenvironment against drug-induced apoptosis through induction of survival signaling pathways such as PI3K/Akt in tumor cells [30, 31].

Measurements of some enzyme activities that take part in inflammatory processes may be useful in differential diagnosis between benign and malignant ascites. Expressions of cyclo-oxygenase-2 mRNA in benign and malignant ascites of different etiologies (liver, stomach, bladder, ovary) showed higher values in malignant than in benign ascites in the ratio of 42.9%:6.7%. In ovarian cancer, the proportion of this marker in the malignant ascites was the highest (57.1%), whereas in malignant ascites of other localizations, it was 33–40% [32].

Apart from measuring immunological and inflammatory reactions in blood, ascites, and tumor surroundings and assessing lymphocyte, macrophages, specific enzymes, NK cells, and other elements of the immune response, it is also very important to demonstrate cytokines, chemokines, and specific protein factors between the immune system communication and tumor cells. Concentration of proinflammatory cytokines in ascites is 40–500 folds higher than in serum [33].

Malignant ascites can be described as a dynamic reservoir of survival factors, including cytokines, chemokines, and growth factors, that individually or in combination suppress immune response and tumor cell growth and progression. An analysis of the ascites from a few epithelial cancers showed increased expression of several factors, including angiogenin, angiopoietin, IL-6, IL-6R, IL-8, IL-10, leptin, MCP-1, MIF, NAP-2, osteoprotegerin (OPG), and urokinase plasminogen activator receptor (uPAR) [34].

OPG has been known as a product of mesothelial and endothelial cell secretion, promoting tumor growth and angiogenesis and inhibiting TRAIL-induced apoptosis of ovarian cancer cells induced by TNF [35]. This is what differentiates benign from malignant ascites, since mesothelial cells in malignant ascites can produce factors that disable the impact of apoptotic TNF factor on malignant cells of ovarian cancer. Such a production is genetic in origin. Further analyses of gene expression in stimulating mesothelial cells of malignant ascites showed that 484 genes were upregulated and 165 genes were downregulated. Genes associated with the regulation of cell growth and proliferation, cell death, and organization have higher gene expression. Top networks upregulated by malignant ascites included Akt and NF-κB survival pathways.

Leptin is an adipokine predominately produced by adipocytes and promotes ovarian cancer cell growth *in vitro* [36].

Ascites of malignant potential constitutes a microenvironment that stimulates production of integrins in epithelial-mesenchymal ovarian cancer cells. These integrins assist the formation of two invasive phenotypes for migration and formation of malignant cells in spheroid structure.

Out of other already mentioned factors elevated in malignant ascites, IL-10 is worth mentioning. This interleukin may help tumor cells to evade host immunological surveillance. Its immunological suppressive activity is known to inhibit T helper cell proliferation, impede dendritic cell maturation, and inhibit T cells co-stimulatory molecules [37–39].

Consistent with that, ascites-derived ovarian tumor cells have been shown to constitutively release CD95 ligand (also known as Fas ligand), which can induce apoptosis in immune cells expressing CD95 [40].

The factors presented in the malignant ascites may also have a negative impact on natural killer T (NKT) cell activity, since GD3 ganglioside contained in ascites inhibits killer T (NKT) cell activity and the interaction of ovarian cancer cells with natural killer cells, thus protecting ovarian cancer cells from host immunity [41].

There is also a correlation between regulatory T cells (Treg) (which inhibit tumor-specific T-cell immunity) in the ascites and reduced survival in patients with ovarian cancer [42].

Besides aforementioned IL-10, the concentration of other inflammatory cytokines, such as IL-1β, IL-6, and IL-8, is significantly higher in the ascites than in the serum. Increased concentration of these interleukins due to immunosuppressive and tumorigenic effect correlates with poor prognosis and response to therapy or chemoresistance [43, 44].

Special attention should be paid to IL-6 whose increased presence in the malignant ascites promotes tumor growth, migration, and invasion, but facilitates chemoresistance [39, 40] and angiogenesis. So, high level of IL-6 is an independent predictor of patient's response to therapy [45–48].

Furthermore, ascites from ovarian cancer patients containing elevated levels of IL-1 was correlated with increased overall survival [49].

Hepatocyte growth factor in malignant ascites stimulates the migration of ovarian cancer cells [50].

Lysophosphatidic acid (LPA), a bioactive phospholipid present in high levels in the ascites of ovarian cancer patients and produced by ovarian cancer cells, with increased transcriptional regulation of vascular endothelial growth factor (VEGF), uPA, IL-6, and IL-8 affects membrane permeability and encourages ascites accumulation [51, 52].

The VEGF concentration is significantly higher in the ascites than in the serum, confirming increased angiogenic activity of the peritoneal cavity. The role of VEGF in the production of ascites is based on the increased permeability of peritoneal membranes and downregulation of tight junction protein claudin 5 and on the induction of tyrosine phosphorylation of cadherin-catenin complex, resulting in decreased endothelial junctional strength and increased permeability of the blood vessels. Neoangiogenesis and increased permeability of the peritoneal and endothelial membrane synergistically form the ascites [53, 54]. VEGF increases the permeability of venules and small veins for plasma proteins with a potency 10,000 times higher than histamine [55]. Besides a role in the pathogenesis of ascites, VEGF results in reduced effects of antiapoptotic bcl-2 protein and decreases sensitivity to chemotherapy and radiation therapy. Similar effects and chemoresistance are obtained by other vascular endogenous factors, such as endothelin-1.

Of other prognostic factors to be determined in the ascites, concentration of E-cadherin is distinguished. Its expression is most commonly lost in metastasis, but it is enhanced in the cells from chemoresistant recurrent ovarian tumors, resulting in tumor cells aggregation with limited drug penetration and in decreased susceptibility to chemotherapy [56–58].

As for immunological prognostic factors, a CD4/CD8 T cell ratio in ascites and the presence of Treg are of considerable importance. High T cell/Treg ratio independently predicts increased survival [59].

On the other hand, reduced accumulation of CD3+CD56+ cells (natural killer or natural killer-like T cells) in the ascites is always correlated with poor prognosis, because it is present in patients with increased platinum resistance [60].

Proinflammatory cytokines in ascites are directly associated with tumor cells phenotype and promotion of human mesothelial cells. Hepatocyte growth factor (HGF) and epidermal growth factor (EGF) are migration mediators of cancer-associated peritoneal mesothelial cells by activating cMet and possibly downstream ERK1/2 and Akt pathways. Thus, ascites not only stimulates tumor growth but also its migration and metastatic growth [61].

Ascitic fluid has been proven to contain other chemokines and chemokine receptors as well, such as CXCR3, that support migration and metastatic progression of malignant cells by triggering the migration of cancer cells along the peritoneal cavity. Increased expression of this chemokine is associated with a higher stage of the disease and positive lymph nodes. In future, this chemokine could be considered a factor of targeted therapy [62].

Besides aforementioned migration factors found in ascites, there is also vascular cell adhesion molecule-1 (VCAM-1). Its elevation in the ascites and the serum is associated with increased risk of malignant cell metastasis [63].

Ascites may also increase migration and metastatic progression by weakening the factors that cause a potential metastatic blockade by affecting TGF-β. Environmental and local factors in the ascites promote migration of malignant cells by repressing miRNA-125b. Repression of miRNA-125b under the influence of local factors stimulates metastatic progression in the ascites by the influence of TGF-β [64].

Some adipokines found in the ascitic fluid can also affect migration and metastatic progression. Visfatin is a novel adipokine exhibiting high levels in many types of carcinomas. Elevated levels of visfatin in ascites are associated with ovarian cancer intraperitoneal dissemination. Some recent studies have shown that ascites-derived visfatin promoted migration of ovarian cancer cells through Rho/ROCK signaling-mediated actin polymerization, which was required for ovarian cancer intraperitoneal dissemination. These studies are important in terms of potential future recommendations regarding ovarian cancer targeted therapy [65].

Immunosuppressive microenvironment in ascites influences not only the number of specific lymphocytes and immune response factors but also their functionality as well. A study that analyzed functional characteristics of specific lymphocytes, Treg lymphocytes, NK cells, TNF cells, and specific cytokines in ascites associated with malignant cells and in ascites without malignant cells showed that functional ability of NK cells is reduced in malignant ascites.

Functional ability of NK cells was determined indirectly by measuring the concentration of CD 107 marker, which shows the degree of degranulation and efficacy of NK cells. In ascites with malignant cells compared to ascites without malignant cells, CD 107 concentration is lower both with and without direct stimulation by IL 2, due to pronounced immunosuppressive effect of tumor microenvironment. On the other hand, the concentration of local inflammatory factors of TNF and TREG cells is greater in malignant ascites [66].

Ascites inhibits T lymphocyte function as well. Inhibition of T-cell receptor-induced nuclear factor-kappa B (NF-κB) and nuclear factor of activated T-cell (NFAT) signaling in tumor-associated T cells has been proved. This function of T cells is restored in the absence of ascites and when there is no contact with T-lymphocytes [67].

Tumor-associated macrophages (TAMs) are essential for cancer progression. The analyses of TAM in different ovarian cancers suggest that different activities are associated with specific cytokines activation. Activation of IL-6 and IL-10 is associated with increased aggressiveness of ovarian cancer, whereas the activation of IFN-γ is able to neutralize the suppressive effect of ascites on IL-12 expression, a key determinant of a cytotoxic immune response. Cytokines in malignant ascites are generally said to present a mixture of protumorigenic and antitumorigenic factors that form a unique microenvironment. Protumorigenic cytokines, including IL-6, IL-8, IL-10, IL-15, IP-10, MCP-1, MIP-1β, and vascular endothelial growth factor (VEGF), and significantly reduced levels of IL-2, IL-5, IL-7, and IL-17 result in the formation of proinflammatory and immunosuppressive tumor microenvironment [33].

Of all aforementioned cytokines, IL-6 and IL-10 concentration deserves special attention, since increased concentration of these cytokines is a bad prognostic parameter associated with poor response to therapy. The concentration of these proinflammatoy cytokines in ascites is 40–500 folds greater than in serum. IL-6 may be secreted in ovarian cancer cells, tumor-associated macrophages, and peritoneal mesothelial cells, which have the highest potential for secretion of this interleukin [68, 69].

An algorithm, including the concentration of aforementioned IL-6 and IL-10, as well as the concentration of leptin and CA 125 markers, is a good prognostic parameter of tumor progression and resistance to first-line therapy [28].

A lot of studies have confirmed that the association between the processes of coagulation and inflammation can be proved in oncologic patients. In this regard, it has been proved that thrombin as a central factor of coagulation may have an important role in the regulation of inflammatory response. A lot of studies have confirmed that thrombin-like activity in ovarian cancer-associated ascites may result in modulation of multiple cytokines network. On the other hand, the anticoagulant antithrombin reverses and prevents IL-12 inhibition induced by ascites. The use of specific thrombin receptors (PAR) agonist peptides has proved that IL-12 inhibition is thrombin-specific and dependent. These data suggest that there is a relationship between IL-12 concentration and coagulation, where thrombin is the key enzyme in IL-12 inhibition. This inhibition is the most important in forming the tumor microenvironment that enables the escape of immune system effects on tumorogenesis [70].

http://dx.doi.org/10.5772/intechopen.70476

The acellular fraction of ascitic fluid in ovarian cancer is an environment that promotes *de novo* resistance of tumor cells by producing protective microenvironment that contributes to tumor cell growth and disease recurrence. Environmental factors of ascites inhibit drug- and death receptor-induced apoptosis. The use of enzyme-linked immunosorbent assay (ELISA) for measuring IL-6 and IL-8 levels in the ascites determined that the level of these cytokines correlates with clinical and pathological parameters and progression-free survival, suggesting that elevated IL-6 is an independent predictor of shorter progression-free survival [71].

7. Malignant ascites—cellular factors

The origin and phenotype of the cells in the ascites is poorly understood. Ascites contains a complex heterogeneous mixture of resident and nonresident cell populations, each population of cells has a specific role and both populations interact with each other through soluble mediators. The resident components of the ascites include tumor cells, stromal cells, and cancer-associated fibroblasts (CAF), whereas cells recruited from the outside of the tumor environment, including infiltrating macrophages/monocytes, bone marrow-derived mesenchymal stem cells (MSC), and cytotoxic or Treg, belong to nonresident populations.

Cancer-associated fibroblasts (CAFs) are important in the autocrine-paracrine promotion, proliferation, and migration of cancer cells [72].

Similar effect on tumor progression is also attributed to human peritoneal mesothelial cells (HPMC) [73, 74]. Lysophosphatidic acid (LPA) produced by HPMC increases adhesion, migration, and invasion of ovarian cancer cells [74]. On the other hand, cancer-associated mesothelial cells have been proven to produce factors that stimulate chemoresistance in ovarian cancer cells [75]. In a response to exposure to malignant ascites, HPMC also produce dipeptidyl peptidase IV and VEGF [76, 77].

Ascitic tumor cells may be presented as individual adherent cells and as aggregates of nonadherent cells known as spheroids [78]. Spheroids have low levels of E-cadherin, express epithelial cell adhesion molecule (EpCAM) and cytokeratin, and have a pronounced ability of invasion and recurrence and a more rapid occurrence of ascites. This type of malignant cells with the aggregates is chemoresistant due to limited drug penetration through these multicellular cell aggregates [79, 80]. These spheroid cells mimic traits of cancer stem cells (CSC). CSCs are cell population resistant to chemotherapy and are a source of proliferating tumor cells with progressive differentiation potential.

Further evidence of spheroid aggregates showed that there are two subtypes of adherent cells—those with mesenchymal-like and epithelial-like morphology. Both types are similar to stem/progenitor cells that have a potential for self-renewal and the expression of cancer stem cells, including $CD44^{high}$, $CD24^{low}$, and $AC133^{+}$ [81]. These cells also express genes responsible for tumorigenesis and metastasis: BMP-2, BMP4, TGF-β, EGFR, and integrin $\alpha_2 \beta_1$ [23]. Future studies should be directed to these nonadherent spheroidal cell aggregates due to their role in carcinogenesis and metastatic progression.

The stromal cellular components of ascites include fibroblasts, endothelial or mesothelial cells, adipocytes, adipose tissue-derived stromal cells, bone marrow-derived stem cells, and immune cells [82, 83]. Stromal cells activate angiogenesis and growth factor and play an important role in malignant progression.

8. Metabolic and biochemical parameters of communication between cellular and acellular factors

The analysis of metabolites, chemical compounds, and metabolic profile in malignant ascites in comparison to benign ascites (cirrhosis) showed the difference in fatty acids, cholesterol, ceramide, glycerol-3-phosphate, glucose, and glucose-3-phosphate. 2-Hydroxyisovalerate is the least present metabolite, but glucose-1-phosphate (G1P) is the dominant metabolite in the malignant ascites. 2-Hydroxyisovalerate is a product of amino acids breakdown and is elevated in patients with ketoacidosis. G1P is a product of glycogenolysis suggesting an increase of glucose breakdown and increased metabolism.

Furthermore, glucose transporter (GLUT) 1 or GLUT3 and glycolytic enzymes, hexokinase (HK) II, are overexpressed in several tumor cells and suggested to be an indicator of poor prognosis in different malignancies, including ovarian cancer [84]. Overexpression of hexokinase (HK) II is associated with the disease progression and chemoresistance [85]. Additionally, glycolate, glucose, furanose, and fructose are significantly decreased, whereas glycerol-3-phosphate, cholesterol, ceramide, and monoacylglycerol (MAG; 18:0/0:0/0:0) are significantly increased in EOC patient-derived ascites [86]. Moreover, ceramide, derivatives of fatty acids, and LPA are identified only in malignant ascites [86].

Biochemical analyses of proteins in ascites of benign etiology identified about 1855 types of protein and in malignant ascites 2096 proteins. About 424 proteins were identified as specific to malignant ascites [87]. The concentration of pyruvate kinase isozymes M1/M2 (PKM1/2), glyceraldehyde phosphate dehydrogenase (GAPDH), and mesothelin (MSLN) was elevated in comparison to benign ascites. The most specific differences between these two types of ascites regarding protein occurrence were up to sevenfolds in RNA components.

Malignant ascites also exhibits higher concentration of complex glycans, unlike benign ascites that contains simple glycans. A complex N-Glycan analysis of ascitic fluids showed highly fucosylated and sialylated complex and hybrid glycans. Other protein components specific to malignant ascites include annexin, mucin, and peroxiredoxin families [88].

In malignant ascites also are an abundance of other biochemical components, including N, haptoglobin, fibronectin, lumican, fibulin, hemopexin, ceruloplasmin, alpha-1-antitrypsin, alpha-1-antichymotrypsin, and clusterin, hemopexin, and fibulin glycopeptides [89].

Exosomes in ascites—Exosomes size in malignant ascites is in the range between 30 and 100 nm in diameter. Inward budding of the late endosomal membrane to segregate the cargos, including lipids, proteins, and nucleic acids, within the membrane-covered vesicles is responsible for their formation [90]. Molecular signatures of donor cells having the ability to circulate throughout the body and potentially transferring information between cells to alter gene expression in recipient cells have been identified in exosomes [91]. Furthermore, it has been determined that exosome-derived molecular cargos contain distinct subsets of disease-specific biomarkers, including miR-200c, miR-214, CA125, Muc-1, and CD24 [92].

The level of 9 of 10 tested agents (CCL2, CXCL1, CXCL5, CXCL8, CXCL12, HGF, PAI-1, TGF-β1, and VEGF) was found to be the greatest in the fluids from undifferentiated and advanced cancers, but the concentration of remaining 2 agents (IL-6 and uPA) was the highest in ascites from serous carcinoma [93].

9. Therapeutic approach for the patients with ascites

Primary treatment option in the management of ovarian cancer is cytoreductive surgery and platinum-based therapy with an expected response rate of 70%. However, many women experience recurrence of the disease within 12–18 months, refractory to standard platinum treatment.

Successful treatment of ascites is limited by the fact that the complete pathogenic mechanism is still poorly understood, and on the other hand, the advanced stage of the disease limits the successful management of the disease and quality of life.

Standard therapy of ascites mainly includes repeated paracentesis in more than 96% of cases. This method is effective in rapid control of distressing symptoms, such as dyspnea, orthopnea, pain, and peritoneal content.

Paracentesis is the most commonly used treatment modality in more than 98% of cases. This method is minimally invasive and may be used under ultrasound control, and the relief of symptoms is reported in 78% of cases. First, patients show relief of abdominal bloating and anorexia, then dyspnea, insomnia, and fatigue. Paracentesis is performed by inserting a 14-gauge needle with a 16-gauge catheter. The drainage of more than 9 L increases the risk of intravascular pressure, hypotension, hypovolemia, hypoproteinemia, and electrolytic imbalance [94].

However, this method has its limitations, since more than 5 L of ascitic fluid removal may affect plasma volume and renal function. For these reasons, 5% dextrose infused simultaneously with paracentesis has been advocated. Possible complications of this method also include hypoproteinemia, hypotension, secondary peritonitis, perforation, and pulmonary embolism [95, 96]. In order to prevent possible complications and homeostatic imbalance, it is necessary to perform blood tests control, focusing on protein and electrolyte levels, and the catheter needle should not stay in one site longer than 24 hours. In order to reduce the risk of infection, antibiotic therapy is sometimes used during the first week of treatment after puncture. Courtney et al. [97] reported their results regarding the use of pleurx catheter that could be kept in a patient for 70 days, reducing the incidence and the risk of septic complications.

Serial paracentesis not only provide relief of symptoms but also promote loss of proteins, hypovolemia, and potential spread of cancer cells to site of drainage.

Complications may include pain, perforation, peritonitis, frequent hospitalizations, and corrections of hypoproteinemia and hypoalbuminemia.

Diuretic therapy in the management of the ascites is rarely performed (61% of all ascites) and is less effective than paracentesis (45%) [98]. Unlike benign ascites (liver cirrhosis and congestive heart failure), malignant ascites respond poorly to the therapy including fluid and salt restrictions and diuretics that may cause complications such as a decrease in volume, electrolytic imbalance, and renal dysfunction.

Pockros et al. proved in his paper that renin levels were elevated in patients with hepatic metastases, whereas normal renin levels were confirmed in carcinomatosis without hepatic metastases [99]. Patients without hepatic metastases and with diuretic use had 1 kg/d in weight loss without hypotension, and those without metastases and in carcinomatosis group had 0.5 kg/d in weight loss with hypotension and renal dysfunction.

The most common medical therapeutic approach includes diuretics therapy. Diuretic drugs used in the management of the disease are aldosterone antagonist such as spironolactone at a dose of 100–200 mg daily and furosemide at an initial dosage of 40–80 mg per day [100]. The use of these drugs increases the risk of hypovolemia, hypotension, and renal failure [101], so their usage is allowed, but with a time limit. Contraindications are hyponatremia <125 mmol/l, hepatorenal-related decrease of sodium excretion to <30 mmol/day, renal insufficiency with serum creatinine >1.5 mg/dl, acute encephalopathy, and acute bacterial infection [102]. The use of diuretics also increases the risk of thromboembolic complications due to chemotherapy drug concentrations, and possible additional symptoms include gynecomastia, renal tubular acidosis, and hyperkalemia.

Another palliative attempt to moderate the symptoms of ascites is the application of chemotherapeutics into the peritoneal cavity. This treatment aims at delivering higher concentrations of drugs to the target site and minimizing resorption toxic effects. The intraperitoneal application of cisplatin and paclitaxel cytostatic drugs is most commonly used in the treatment. Complications of this method include infections, pain, blockage or leaks, and abdominal pain. Limiting factors are short-term effects and a maximum of 5 mm penetration into a tumor deposit with limiting effects to existing adhesions. Other side effects include abdominal pain, ileus, peritonitis, abscess, and necrosis.

The attempts to increase the cytotoxicity of cisplatin and paclitaxel in intraperitoneal application resulted in utilization of hyperthermic medium (40.5–43°C). This procedure is called hyperthermic intraperitoneal chemotherapy (HIPEC). The method was approved by Japanese National Insurance in 1981. The results of HIPEC treatment regarding overall survival rate are better in comparison to reduction of ascitic fluid, but without statistically significant difference [101].

Chemotherapy in the management of ascites can be systemic and intraperitoneal. Intraperitoneal chemotherapy has local cytotoxicity 2–3 times higher than systemic one without systemic absorption or cytotoxicity. Hyperthermia (over 39°) increases local cytotoxic effects by inhibiting replication and repair. The best results are achieved directly after the surgery (complete cytoreduction) since fibrin depositions and adhesion formations are thin at that time. Combined modality treatment of surgical procedure and intraperitoneal chemotherapy using cisplatin, bleomycin, and mitomycin C prevents recurrence of ascites in 75% of patients. The fact that patients without positive peritoneal cytology do not develop ascites suggests that cytostatic therapy administration can prevent formation of ascites [103].

Besides intraperitoneal application of cytostatics, other drugs can be used intraperitoneally, such as intraperitoneal tumor necrosis factor (TNF), interferon, vascular endothelial growth factor, and other immunomodulators.

TNF at 0.08–0.014 mg/m^2 diluted in 5% human albumin is applied into the abdomen for 24–48 hours, and the procedure is repeated on the 8th day.

Improvements regarding reduction of ascitic fluid can be seen after three doses, but improvements in mucinous ovarian cancer have not been reported [104].

Intraperitoneal interferon-α (IFN-α) 2b application was described in studies by Sartori et al. [105]. Complete response was achieved in 29.3%, a partial response in 36.6%, and no response in 34.1%. Ovarian cancer patients had the highest global response (65%).

Clinical importance of immunomodulator OK-432 application has been studied. It is a lyophilized powder of *Streptococcus pyogenes*, showing effects only in patients with malignant ascites associated with gastrointestinal-related cancer. Studies of ascites and ovarian cancer are not available [101].

One of the surgical methods used in palliative treatment of ascites is peritoneovenous shunting. Surgical options in treating ascites include peritoneovenous shunts and radical peritonectomy. The first data on peritoneovenous shunts date back to 1974 when LeVeen first introduced it. A modified Denver shunt was developed later. The benefits of this method in comparison to paracentesis include reduced need for repeated paracentesis and maintenance of normal serum albumin concentrations. In malignant ascites, reduction and control of ascites are achieved in 75% of shunts [106]. Patients selected for shunt placement should undergo cardiac and respiratory evaluations.

Faught et al. [107] evaluated some possible complications of this method, such as fever, coagulopathy, infection, and tumor embolization [101]. Contraindications are loculated ascites, portal hypertension, coagulation disorders, elevated bilirubin levels, advanced cardiac or renal failure, hemorrhagic ascites, or fluid protein >4.5 g/l. The study has not proven increased probability of disseminating malignant cells by this treatment modality. What is important is that the application of this shunt showed better clinical results for ascites in ovarian cancer patients than in gastrointestinal cancer patients, in relation 50:15%, respectively. However, the application of shunts is indicated only for patients who cannot benefit from any other treatment and who can profit from it if their life expectancy is long enough. The median survival ranged in the different studies from 52 to 266 days, reflecting the high heterogeneity of patients, and possible fatal complications are pulmonary edema or emboli [96, 108].

Finally, other surgical therapeutic procedures include radical peritonectomy. It is an extensive surgical intervention involving complete removal of the peritoneum combined with intraperitoneal chemotherapy. This is an extensive operation with significant morbidity, although initial results appear to demonstrate that it decreases the production of ascites.

A modern, innovative approach in treating malignant ascites is monoclonal antibody therapy, directed at one of the basic etiological factors of ascites—neoangiogenesis. In that respect, the drugs used, such as anti-vascular endothelial vascular factor (VEGF), may have potential tumor-suppressive effects.

Bevacizumab (Avastin®; Genentech, Inc., South San Francisco, CA) is a recombinant humanized monoclonal antibody to VEGF composed of human IgG_1 framework regions and antigen-binding complementarity-determining regions from a murine antibody that blocks the binding of human VEGF to its receptors [109].

Bevacizumab is a humanized monoclonal antibody directed against VEGF-A as target therapy [110]. After its initial approval by the Food and Drug Administration (FDA) in 2004 for unresectable colorectal cancer, its indication for the treatment of different cancers has been accepted [111, 112]. The trials GOG-0218 and ICON7 reported benefits of this therapy combined with platinum therapy in patients with ovarian cancer. The AURELIA trial studied bevacizumab in combination with non-platinum chemotherapy and proved its success in platinum-resistant ovarian cancer [113]. In 2014, FDA approved bevacizumab for use only in recurrent, platinum-resistant ovarian cancer [114]. In 2016, this drug also received FDA approval for platinum-sensitive recurrent ovarian cancer, based on findings of a large GOG-0213 trial.

Therapeutic application of bevacizumab has also demonstrated significant benefits in patients with recurrent disease and ascites. Most common side effects are neutropenia and thrombocytopenia. Other serious, but rare side effects include gastrointestinal bleeding, thromboembolic events, hypertension, and proteinuria.

The studies analyzing quality of life and the recurrence of the disease in patients with ascites treated with repeated paracentesis and monoclonal anti-vascular drugs have shown that palliative treatment of malignant ascites using paracentesis or combined paracentesis and intraperitoneal chemotherapy negatively impacts patients' health-related quality of life (HRQL) and shortens the disease-free interval. Monoclonal antibody treatment results in better quality of life and in a longer disease-free interval. The median puncture-free survival with catumaxomab is 46 days versus 11 days in the group with paracentesis [115].

Complications of the procedure may be local: shunt occlusion and infections and systemic: DIC (due to coagulation factor dilution, introduction of collagen into the bloodstream), pulmonary edema (9.5–12%), pulmonary embolism (5–7%), and tumor emboli by direct infusion of malignant cells into the bloodstream (3–7%) [116].

Other new therapeutic approaches to be pointed out include immunotherapy with interferon, tumor necrosis factor, Corynebacterium parvum, and Streptococcal preparation OK-432 [117].

10. Conclusion

Due to low symptomatology, a lack of screening, and relatively complicated diagnostic procedures of ovarian carcinoma, more and more women are believed to visit their doctors in advanced stage of the disease, complicated with ascitic fluid.

Cytological findings of ascitic fluid determine the stage of the disease. On the other hand, there is an increasing evidence that peritoneal cytology is a subjective assessment with certain percentage of false-positive and false-negative results that may cause application of unnecessary chemotherapy or nonapplication of necessary chemotherapy. Utilization of available and the development of new immunohistochemical markers should help in increasing sensitivity and specificity of ascitic fluid cytology.

Ascites has unfavorable outcomes and detrimental effects on overall quality of life in affected patients.

The pathophysiology of the incidence of ascites is unclear, complex, and is a combination of increased vascular permeability and obstructed lymphatic drainage.

Because the mechanism of ascites formation is poorly understood, there are no validating guidelines for preventing the formation of ascites. Maximal cytoreductive surgery followed by intraperitoneal or systemic chemotherapy remains to be the gold standard in preventing ascites formation.

Ascites is not only a symptom of a disease but also a specific microenvironment for formation and mediation of protumorigenic signals that control ovarian cancer progression, including proliferation, invasion and anti-apoptosis, chemoresistance, and tumor heterogeneity. Acellular cytokines, protein, and immunological factors influence ovarian cancer progression and its ability to prevent immune responses of the body and tumor reaction to chemotherapy. On the other hand, ascites contributes to disease dissemination, changing its course, and final outcomes.

Management of patients with ascites and ovarian carcinoma is complex, with additional recurrences, and often the goal of the treatment is to target palliative procedures that necessitate hospital environment.

Multidisciplinary approach is necessary in the management of patients and includes not only a gynecologist but also an anesthesiologist, gastroenterologist, surgeon, oncologist, chemotherapist, palliative care doctor, and an oncology pharmacist.

In order to improve overall quality of life and survival of these patients, further investigations of new drugs, monoclonal antibodies, and immunomodulators are needed aiming at prolonged periods between relapses.

Author details

Radomir Živadinović[1]*, Aleksandra Petrić[1], Dane Krtinić[2], Sonja Pop-Trajković Dinić[1] and Biljana Živadinović[3]

*Address all correspondence to: zivadinovicrasa@gmail.com

1 Clinic for Gynecology and Obstetrics, Clinical Center Niš, Faculty of Medicine, Department for Gynecology and Obstetrics, University of Niš, Niš, Serbia

2 Clinic for Oncology, Clinical Center Niš, Faculty of Medicine, University of Niš, Niš, Serbia

3 Clinic for Neurology, Clinical Center Niš, Faculty of Medicine, University of Niš, Niš, Serbia

References

[1] Runyon BA. Care of patients with ascites. New England Journal of Medicine. 1994;**330**(5):337-342. DOI: 10.1056/NEJM199402033300508

[2] Sangisetty SL, Miner TJ. Malignant ascites: A review of prognostic factors, pathophysiology and therapeutic measures. World Journal of Gastrointestinal Surgery. 2012;**4**(4):87-95. DOI: 10.4240/wjgs.v4.i4.87

[3] Becker G, Galandi D, Blum HE. Malignant ascites: Systematic review and guideline for treatment. European Journal of Cancer. 2006;**42**(5):589-597. DOI: 10.1016/j.ejca.2005.11.018

[4] Adam RA, Adam YG. Malignant ascites: Past, present, and future. Journal of the American College of Surgeons. 2004;**198**(6):999-1011. DOI: 10.1016/j.jamcollsurg.2004.01.035

[5] Fukuo Y, Shinohara H, Matsuda T. The distribution of lymphatic stomata in the diaphragm of the golden hamster. Journal of Anatomy. 1990;**169**:13-21

[6] Stanojević Z, Rančić G, Radić S, Potić-Zećević N, Djordjević B, Marković M et al. Pathogenesis of malignant ascites in ovarian cancer patients. Archives of Oncology. 2004;**12**(2):115-118

[7] Garrison RN, Kaelin LD, Galloway RH, Heuser LS. Malignant ascites. Clinical and experimental observations. Annals of Surgery. 1986;**203**(6):644-651

[8] Shen-Gunther J, Mannel RS. Ascites as a predictor of ovarian malignancy. Gynecologic Oncology. 2002;**87**(1):77-83. DOI: 10.1006/gyno.2002.6800

[9] Mackey JR, Venner PM. Malignant ascites: Demographics, therapeutic efficacy and predictors of survival. Canadian Journal of Oncology. 1996;**6**(2):474-480

[10] Lin O. Challenges in the interpretation of peritoneal cytologic specimens. Archives of Pathology and Laboratory Medicine. 2009;**133**(5):739-742. DOI: 10.1043/1543-2165-133.5.739

[11] Zivadinovic R, Petric A, Krtinic D, Stevanovic Milosevic J, Pop Trajkovic Dinic S. Ascites in ovarian carcinoma—Reliability and limitations of cytological analysis. West Indian Med Journal. 2015;**64**(3):236-240. DOI: 10.7727/wimjopen.2014.230

[12] Runyon BA, Hoefs JC, Morgan TR. Ascitic fluid analysis in malignancy-related ascites. Hepatology. 1988;**8**(5):1104-1109. DOI: 10.1002/hep.1840080521

[13] Cheng L, Wolf NG, Rose PG, Rodriguez M, Abdul-Karim FW. Peritoneal washing cytology of ovarian tumors of low malignant potential: Correlation with surface ovarian involvement and peritoneal implants. Acta Cytologica. 1998;**42**(5):1091-1094

[14] Zuna RE, Behrens A. Peritoneal washing cytology in gynecologic cancers: Long-term follow-up of 355 patients. Journal of the National Cancer Institute. 1996;**88**(14):980-987

[15] Karoo RO, Lloyd TD, Garcea G, Redway HD, Robertson GS. How valuable is ascitic cytology in the detection and management of malignancy. Postgrade Medical Journal. 2003;**79**(931):292-294. DOI: 10.1136/pmj.79.931.292

[16] Sirop S, Kanaan M, Wiese D, Dutt N, Karla V, Singh T, et al. A second peritoneal cytology as a prognostic factor in epithelial ovarian cancer. Journal of Clinical Oncology. 2011;**29**:e15558

[17] Hecht JL, Pinkus JL, Pinkus GS. Monoclonal antibody MOC-31 reactivity as a marker for adenocarcinoma in cytologic preparations. Cancer. 2006;**108**(1):56-59. DOI: 10.1002/cncr.21426

[18] Duggan BD, Roman LD, Muderspach LI. Detection of ovarian cancer cells: Comparison of a telomerase assay and cytologic examination. Oxford Journals Medicine. 1998;**90**(3): 238-242

[19] Zhu FL, Ling AS, Wei Q, Ma J, Lu G. Tumor markers in serum and ascites in the diagnosis of benign and malignant ascites. Asian Pacific Journal of Cancer Prevention. 2015;**16**(2):719-722. DOI: 10.7314/APJCP.2015.16.2.719

[20] Latifi A, Luwor RB, Bilandzic M, Nazaretian S, Stenvers K, Pyman J, et al. Isolation and characterization of tumor cells from the ascites of ovarian cancer patients: Molecular phenotype of chemoresistant ovarian tumors. PLoS One. 2012;**7**(10):e46858. DOI: 10.1371/journal.pone.0046858

[21] Rafehi S, Ramos Valdes Y, Bertrand M, McGee J, Préfontaine M, Sugimoto A, et al. TGFβ signaling regulates epithelial–mesenchymal plasticity in ovarian cancer ascites-derived spheroids. Endocrine-Related Cancer. 2016;**23**(3):147-159. DOI: 10.1530/ERC-15-0383

[22] Slack-Davis JK, Atkins KA, Harrer C, Hershey ED, Conaway M. Vascular cell adhesion molecule-1 is a regulator of ovarian cancer peritoneal metastasis. Cancer Research. 2009;**69**(4):1469-1476. DOI: 10.1158/0008-5472.CAN-08-2678

[23] Rizvi I, Gurkan UA, Tasoglu S, Alagic N, Celli JP, Mensah LB, et al. Flow induces epithelial-mesenchymal transition, cellular heterogeneity and biomarker modulation in 3D ovarian cancer nodules. Proceedings of National Academy of Sciences of United States of America. 2013;**110**(22):E1974-E1983. DOI: 10.1073/pnas.1216989110

[24] Buy JN, Moss AA, Ghossain MA, Sciot C, Malbec L, Vadrot D, et al. Peritoneal implants from ovarian tumors: CT findings. Radiology. 1988;**169**(3):691-694. DOI: 10.1148/radiology.169.3.3186993

[25] Kipps E, Tan D, Kaye S. Meeting the challenge of ascites in ovarian cancer: New avenues for therapy and research. Nature Reviews Cancer. 2013;**13**:273-282. DOI: 10.1038/nrc3432

[26] Ahmed N, Stenvers K. Getting to know ovarian cancer ascites: Opportunities for targeted therapy-based transitional research. Frontiers in Oncology. 2013;**3**:256. DOI: 10.3389/fonc.2013.00256

[27] Huang QT, Zhou L, Zeng WJ, Ma QQ, Wang W, Zhong M, et al. Prognostic significance of neutrophil-to-lymphocyte ratio in ovarian cancer: A systematic review and meta-analysis of observational studies. Cellular Physiology and Biochemistry. 2017;**41**(6):2411-2418. DOI: 10.1159/000475911

[28] Lu Y, Huang S, Li P, Chen B, Liu W, Chen Z, et al. Prognostic evaluation of preoperative serum C-reactive protein concentration in patients with epithelial ovarian cancer. Experimental and Therapeutic Medicine. 2015;**9**(5):2003-2007. DOI:10.3892/etm.2015.2350

[29] Lukesova S, Vroblova V, Tosner J, Kopecky J, Sedlakova I, Čermáková E, et al. Comparative study of various subpopulations of cytotoxic cells in blood and ascites from patients with ovarian carcinoma. Contemporary Oncology (Poznan). 2015;**19**(4):290-299. DOI: 10.5114/wo.2015.54388

[30] Lane D, Robert V, Grondin R, Rancourt C, Piche A. Malignant ascites protect against TRAIL-induced apoptosis by activating the PI3K/Akt pathway in human ovarian carcinoma cells. International Journal of Cancer. 2007;**121**(6):1227-1237. DOI: 10.1002/ijc.22840

[31] Lane D, Goncharenko-Khaider N, Rancourt C, Piche A. Ovarian cancer ascites protects from TRAIL-induced cell death through alphavbeta5 integrin-mediated focal adhesion kinase and Akt activation. Oncogene. 2010;**29**(24):3519-3531. DOI: 10.1038/onc.2010.107

[32] Lu J, Li XF, Kong LX, Ma L, Liao SH, Jiang CY. Expression and significance of cyclooxygenase-2 mRNA in benign and malignant ascites. World Journal of Gastroenterology. 2013;**19**(40):6883-6887. DOI: 10.3748/wjg.v19.i40.6883

[33] Giuntoli RL, Webb TJ, Zoso A, Rogers O, Diaz-Montes TP, Bristow RE, et al. Ovarian cancer-associated ascites demonstrates altered immune environment: Implications for antitumor immunity. Anticancer Research. 2009;**29**(8):2875-2884

[34] Matte I, Lane D, Laplante C, Rancourt C, Piche A. Profiling of cytokines in human epithelial ovarian cancer ascites. American Journal of Cancer Research. 2012;**2**(5):566-580

[35] Lane D, Matte I, Rancourt C, Piche A. Osteoprotegerin (OPG) protects ovarian cancer cells from TRAIL-induced apoptosis but does not contribute to malignant ascites-mediated attenuation of TRAIL-induced apoptosis. Journal of Ovarian Research. 2012;**5**(1):34. DOI: 10.1186/1757-2215-5-34

[36] Choi JH, Park SH, Leung PC, Choi KC. Expression of leptin receptors and potential effects of leptin on the cell growth and activation of mitogen-activated protein kinases in ovarian cancer cells. Journal of Clinical Endocrinology and Metabolism. 2005;**90**(1):207-210. DOI: 10.1210/jc.2004-0297

[37] Mocellin S, Wang E, Marincola FM. Cytokines and immune response in the tumor microenvironment. Journal of Immunotherapy. 2001;**24**(5):392-407

[38] Moser M. Dendritic cells in immunity and tolerance-do they display opposite functions? Immunity. 2003;**19**(1):5-8. DOI: 10.1016/S1074-7613(03)00182-1

[39] Moore KW, de Waal Malefyt R, Coffman RL, O'Garra A. Interleukin-10 and the interleukin-10 receptor. Annual Review of Immunology. 2001;**19**:683-765. DOI: 10.1146/annurev.immunol.19.1.683

[40] Abrahams VM, Straszewski SL, Kamsteeg M, Hanczaruk B, Schwartz PE, Rutherford TJ, et al. Epithelial ovarian cancer cells secrete functional Fas ligand. Cancer Research. 2003;**63**(17):5573-5581

[41] Gubbels JA, Felder M, Horibata S, Belisle JA, Kapur A, Holden H, et al. MUC16 provides immune protection by inhibiting synapse formation between NK and ovarian tumor cells. Molecular Cancer. 2010;**9**:11. DOI: 10.1186/1476-4598-9-11

[42] Tan DS, Agarwal R, Kaye SB. Mechanisms of transcoelomic metastasis in ovarian cancer. Lancet Oncology. 2006;**7**(11):925-934. DOI: 10.1016/S1470-2045(06)70939-1

[43] Kryczek I, Grybos M, Karabon L, Klimczak A, Lange A. IL-6 production in ovarian carcinoma is associated with histiotype and biological characteristics of the tumour and influences local immunity. British Journal of Cancer. 2000;**82**(3):621-628. DOI: 10.1054/bjoc.1999.0973

[44] Penson RT, Kronish K, Duan Z, Feller AJ, Stark P, Cook SE, et al. Cytokines IL-1beta, IL-2, IL-6, IL-8, MCP-1, GM-CSF and TNFalpha in patients with epithelial ovarian cancer and their relationship to treatment with paclitaxel. International Journal of Gynecological Cancer. 2000;**10**(1):33-41

[45] Obata NH, Tamakoshi K, Shibata K, Kikkawa F, Tomoda Y. Effects of interleukin-6 on in vitro cell attachment, migration and invasion of human ovarian carcinoma. Anticancer Research. 1997;**17**(1A):337-342

[46] Syed V, Ulinski G, Mok SC, Ho SM. Reproductive hormone-induced, STAT3-mediated interleukin 6 action in normal and malignant human ovarian surface epithelial cells. Journal of National Cancer Institute. 2002;**94**(8):617-629

[47] Wang Y, Niu XL, Qu Y, Wu J, Zhu YQ, Sun WJ, et al. Autocrine production of interleukin-6 confers cisplatin and paclitaxel resistance in ovarian cancer cells. Cancer Letters. 2010;**295**(1):110-123. DOI: 10.1016/j.canlet.2010.02.019

[48] Cohen S, Bruchim I, Graiver D, Evron Z, Oron-Karni V, Pasmanik-Chor M, et al. Platinum-resistance in ovarian cancer cells is mediated by IL-6 secretion via the increased expression of its target cIAP-2. Journal of Molecular Medicine (Berlin). 2013;**91**(3):357-368. DOI: 10.1007/s00109-012-0946-4.

[49] Kryczek I, Banerjee M, Cheng P, Vatan L, Szeliga W, Wei S, et al. Phenotype, distribution, generation, and functional and clinical relevance of Th17 cells in the human tumor environments. Blood. 2009;**114**(6):1141-1149. DOI: 10.1182/blood-2009-03-208249

[50] Sowter HM, Corps AN, Smith SK. Hepatocyte growth factor (HGF) in ovarian epithelial tumour fluids stimulates the migration of ovarian carcinoma cells. International Journal of Cancer. 1999;**83**(4):476-480

[51] Fang X, Yu S, Bast RC, Liu S, Xu HJ, Hu SX, et al. Mechanisms for lysophosphatidic acid-induced cytokine production in ovarian cancer cells. Journal of Biological Chemistry. 2004;**279**(10):9653-9661. DOI: 10.1074/jbc.M306662200

[52] Hu YL, Tee MK, Goetzl EJ, Auersperg N, Mills GB, Ferrara N, et al. Lysophosphatidic acid induction of vascular endothelial growth factor expression in human ovarian cancer cells. Journal of National Cancer Institute. 2001;**93**(10):762-810

[53] Herr D, Sallmann A, Bekes I, Konrad R, Holzheu I, Kreienberg R, et al. VEGF induces ascites in ovarian cancer patients via increasing peritoneal permeability by down-regulation of Claudin 5. Gynecologic Oncology. 2012;**127**(1):210-216. DOI: 10.1016/j.ygyno.2012.05.002

[54] Esser S, Lampugnani MG, Corada M, Dejana E, Risau W. Vascular endothelial growth factor induces VE-cadherin tyrosine phosphorylation in endothelial cells. Journal of Cellular Science. 1998;**111**(Pt 13):1853-1865

[55] Senger DR, Galli SJ, Dvorak AM, Perruzzi CA, Harvey VS, Dvorak HF. Tumor cells secrete a vascular permeability factor that promotes accumulation of ascites fluid. Science. 1983;**219**(4587):983-985

[56] Kosaka N, Hasegawa K, Kiuchi K, Ochiai S, Nagai T, Machida H, et al. Cytological findings of ascitic fluid with a malignant ovarian steroid cell tumor: A case report and literature review. Acta Cytologica. 2017;**61**(2):165-171. DOI: 10.1159/000458750

[57] Ahmed N, Abubaker K, Findlay J, Quinn M. Epithelial mesenchymal transition and cancer stem cell-like phenotypes facilitate chemoresistance in recurrent ovarian cancer. Current Cancer Drug Targets. 2010;**10**(3):268-278

[58] Desoize B, Jardillier J. Multicellular resistance: A paradigm for clinical resistance? Critical Reviews in Oncology Hematology. 2000;**36**(2-3):193-207. DOI: 10.1016/S1040-8428(00)00086-X

[59] Leffers N, Gooden MJ, de Jong RA, Hoogeboom BN, ten Hoor KA, Hollema H, et al. Prognostic significance of tumor-infiltrating T-lymphocytes in primary and metastatic lesions of advanced stage ovarian cancer. Cancer Immunology, Immunotherapy. 2009;**58**(3):449-591. DOI: 10.1007/s00262-008-0583-5

[60] Bamias A, Tsiatas ML, Kafantari E, Liakou C, Rodolakis A, Voulgaris Z, et al. Significant differences of lymphocytes isolated from ascites of patients with ovarian cancer compared to blood and tumor lymphocytes. Association of CD3+CD56+ cells with platinum resistance. Gynecological Oncology. 2007;**106**(1):75-81. DOI: 10.1016/j.ygyno.2007.02.029

[61] Matte I, Lane D, Laplante C, Garde-Granger P, Rancourt C, Piché A. Ovarian cancer ascites enhance the migration of patient-derived peritoneal mesothelial cells via cMet pathway through HGF-dependent and -independent mechanisms. International Journal of Cancer. 2015;**137**(2):289-298. DOI: 10.1002/ijc.29385

[62] Windmüller C, Zech D, Avril S, Boxberg M, Dawidek T, Schmalfeldt B, et al. CXCR3 mediates ascites-directed tumor cell migration and predicts poor outcome in ovarian cancer patients. Oncogenesis. 2017;**6**(5):e331. DOI: 10.1038/oncsis.2017.29

[63] Jakimovska M, Cerne K, Verdenik I, Kobal B. Circulating serum sVCAM-1 concentration in advanced ovarian cancer patients: Correlation with concentration in ascites. Radiology and Oncology. 2014;**48**(3):307-313. DOI: 10.2478/raon-2013-0066

[64] Adhikary T, Wortmann A, Finkernagel F, Lieber S, Nist A, Stiewe T, et al. Interferon signaling in ascites-associated macrophages is linked to a favorable clinical outcome in a subgroup of ovarian carcinoma patients. BMC Genomics. 2017;**18**(1):243. DOI: 10.1186/s12864-017-3630-9

[65] Li Y, Li X, Liu KR, Zhang JN, Liu Y, Zhu Y. Visfatin derived from ascites promotes ovarian cancer cell migration through Rho/ROCK signaling-mediated actin polymerization. European Journal of Cancer Prevention. 2015;**24**(3):231-239. DOI: 10.1097/CEJ.0000000000000064

[66] da Silva RF, Yoshida A, Cardozo DM, Jales RM, Paust S, Derchain S, et al. Natural killer cells response to IL-2 stimulation is distinct between ascites with the presence or absence of malignant cells in ovarian cancer patients. International Journal of Molecular Science. 2017;**18**(5):E856. DOI: 10.3390/ijms18050856

[67] Simpson-Abelson MR, Loyall JL, Lehman HK, Barnas JL, Minderman H, O'Loughlin KL, et al. Human ovarian tumor ascites fluids rapidly and reversibly inhibit T cell receptor-induced NF-kappaB and NFAT signaling in tumor-associated T cells. Cancer Immunology. 2013;**13**:14

[68] Lane D, Matte I, Rancourt C, Piche A. Prognostic significance of IL-6 and IL-8 ascites levels in ovarian cancer patients. BMC Cancer. 2011;**11**:210. DOI: 10.1186/1471-2407-11-210

[69] Lane D, Matte I, Garde-Granger P et al. Inflammation-regulating factors in ascites as predictive biomarkers of drug resistance and progression-free survival in serous epithelial ovarian cancers. BMC Cancer. 2015;**15**:492. DOI: 10.1186/s12885-015-1511-7

[70] Naldini A, Morena E, Belotti D, Carraro F, Allavena P, Giavazzi R. Identification of thrombin-like activity in ovarian cancer associated ascites and modulation of multiple cytokine networks. Thrombosis and Haemostasis. 2011;**106**(4):705-711. DOI: 10.1160/TH11-05-0311

[71] Puiffe ML, Le Page C, Filali-Mouhim A, Zietarska M, Ouellet V, Tonin PN, et al. Characterization of ovarian cancer ascites on cell invasion, proliferation, spheroid formation, and gene expression in an in vitro model of epithelial ovarian cancer. Neoplasia. 2007;**9**(10):820-829

[72] Paraiso KH, Smalley KS. Fibroblast-mediated drug resistance in cancer. Biochemical Pharmacology. 2013;**85**(8):1033-1041. DOI: 10.1016/j.bcp.2013.01.018

[73] Pasquet M, Golzio M, Mery E, Rafii A, Benabbou N, Mirshahi P, et al. Hospicells (ascites-derived stromal cells) promote tumorigenicity and angiogenesis. International Journal of Cancer. 2010;**126**(9):2090-2101. DOI: 10.1002/ijc.24886

[74] Ren J, Xiao YJ, Singh LS, Zhao X, Zhao Z, Feng L, et al. Lysophosphatidic acid is constitutively produced by human peritoneal mesothelial cells and enhances adhesion, migration, and invasion of ovarian cancer cells. Cancer Research. 2006;**66**(6):3006-3014. DOI: 10.1158/0008-5472.CAN-05-1292

[75] Matte I, Lane D, Bachvarov D, Rancourt C, Piche A. Role of malignant ascites on human mesothelial cells and their gene expression profiles. BMC Cancer. 2014;**14**:288. DOI: 10.1186/1471-2407-14-288

[76] Kajiyama H, Kikkawa F, Maeda O, Suzuki T, Ino K, Mizutani S. Increased expression of dipeptidyl peptidase IV in human mesothelial cells by malignant ascites from ovarian carcinoma patients. Oncology. 2002;**63**(2):158-165

[77] Stadlmann S, Amberger A, Pollheimer J, Gastl G, Offner FA, Margreiter R, et al. Ovarian carcinoma cells and IL-1beta-activated human peritoneal mesothelial cells are possible sources of vascular endothelial growth factor in inflammatory and malignant peritoneal effusions. Gynecological Oncology. 2005;**97**(3):784-789. DOI: 10.1016/j.ygyno.2005.02.017

[78] Wintzell M, Hjerpe E, Avall Lundqvist E, Shoshan M. Protein markers of cancer-associated fibroblasts and tumor-initiating cells reveal subpopulations in freshly isolated ovarian cancer ascites. BMC Cancer. 2012;**12**:359. DOI: 10.1186/1471-2407-12-359

[79] Fayad W, Brnjic S, Berglind D, Blixt S, Shoshan MC, Berndtsson M, et al. Restriction of cisplatin induction of acute apoptosis to a subpopulation of cells in a three-dimensional carcinoma culture model. International Journal of Cancer. 2009;**125**(10):2450-2455. DOI: 10.1002/ijc.24627

[80] Tannock IF, Lee CM, Tunggal JK, Cowan DS, Egorin MJ. Limited penetration of anticancer drugs through tumor tissue: A potential cause of resistance of solid tumors to chemotherapy. Clinical Cancer Research. 2002;**8**(3):878-884

[81] Ho CM, Chang SF, Hsiao CC, Chien TY, Shih DT. Isolation and characterization of stromal progenitor cells from ascites of patients with epithelial ovarian adenocarcinoma. Journal of Biomedical Science. 2012;**19**:23. DOI: 10.1186/1423-0127-19-23

[82] Wels J, Kaplan RN, Rafii S, Lyden D. Migratory neighbors and distant invaders: Tumor-associated niche cells. Genes and Development. 2008;**22**(5):559-574. DOI: 10.1101/gad.1636908

[83] Bhowmick NA, Neilson EG, Moses HL. Stromal fibroblasts in cancer initiation and progression. Nature. 2004;**432**(7015):332-337. DOI: 10.1038/nature03096

[84] Carvalho KC, Cunha IW, Rocha RM, Ayala FR, Cajaíba MM, Begnami MD, et al. GLUT1 expression in malignant tumors and its use as an immunodiagnostic marker. Clinics (Sao Paulo). 2011;**66**(6):965-972. DOI: 10.1590/S1807-59322011000600008

[85] Suh DH, Kim MA, Kim H, Kim MK, Kim HS, Chung HH, et al. Association of overexpression of hexokinase II with chemoresistance in epithelial ovarian cancer. Clinical and Experimental Medicine. 2014;**14**(3):345-353. DOI: 10.1007/s10238-013-0250-9

[86] Shender VO, Pavlyukov MS, Ziganshin RH, Arapidi GP, Kovalchuk SI, Anikanov NA, et al. Proteome-metabolome profiling of ovarian cancer ascites reveals novel components involved in intercellular communication. Molecular and Cellular Proteomics. 2014;**13**(12):3558-3571. DOI: 10.1074/mcp.M114.041194

[87] Hartmann D, Lucks J, Fuchs S, Schiffmann S, Schreiber Y, Ferreirós N, et al. Long chain ceramides and very long chain ceramides have opposite effects on human breast and colon cancer cell growth. International Journal of Biochemistry and Cell Biology. 2012;**44**(4):620-628. DOI: 10.1016/j.biocel.2011.12.019

[88] Stuchlíková E, Zahradníková M, Nenutil R, Valík D, Vojtěšek B, Novotný M, et al. Ascites may provide useful information for diagnosis of ovarian cancer. Klinicka Onkologie. 2017;**30**(Suppl 1):187-190

[89] Miyamoto S, Ruhaak LR, Stroble C, Salemi MR, Phinney B, Lebrilla CB, et al. Glycoproteomic analysis of malignant ovarian cancer ascites fluid identifies unusual glycopeptides. Journal of Proteome Research. 2016;**15**(9):3358-3376. DOI: 10.1021/acs.jproteome.6b00548

[90] Guo L, Guo N. Exosomes: Potent regulators of tumor malignancy and potential bio-tools in clinical application. Critical Reviews in Oncology Hematology. 2015;**95**(3):346-358. DOI: 10.1016/j.critrevonc.2015.04.002

[91] Valadi H, Ekstrom K, Bossios A, Sjostrand M, Lee JJ, Lotvall JO. Exosome-mediated transfer of mRNAs and microRNAs is a novel mechanism of genetic exchange between cells. Nature Cell Biology. 2007;**9**(6):654-659. DOI: 10.1038/ncb1596

[92] Taylor DD, Gercel-Taylor C. MicroRNA signatures of tumor-derived exosomes as diagnostic biomarkers of ovarian cancer. Gynecologic Oncology. 2008;**110**(1):13-21. DOI: 10.1016/j.ygyno.2008.04.033

[93] Mikuła-Pietrasik J, Uruski P, Szubert S, Moszyński R, Szpurek D, Sajdak S, et al. Biochemical composition of malignant ascites determines high aggressiveness of undifferentiated ovarian tumors. Medical Oncology. 2016;**33**(8):94. DOI: 10.1007/s12032-016-0810-4

[94] Fischer DS. Abdominal paracentesis for malignant ascites. Archives of Internal Medicine. 1979;**139**(2):235

[95] Stukan M. Drainage of malignant ascites: Patient selection and perspectives. Cancer Management and Research. 2017;**9**:115-130. DOI: 10.2147/CMAR.S100210

[96] Kim S, Kim B, Song YS. Ascites modulates cancer cell behavior, contributing to tumor heterogeneity in ovarian cancer. Cancer Science. 2016;**107**(9):1173-1178. DOI: 10.1111/cas.12987

[97] Courtney AL, Nemcek AA, Rosenberg SM. Efficacy and safety of the pleurx catheter when used to treat recurrent malignant ascites. Journal of Vascular and Interventional Radiology. 2006;**17**(2): S25

[98] Gamblin V, Da Silva A, Villet S, El Hajbi F. Supportive care for malignant ascites in palliative phase: Place of paracentesis and diuretics. Bulletin du Cancer. 2015;**102**(11):940-945. DOI: 10.1016/j.bulcan.2015.09.002

[99] Pockros PJ, Esrason KT, Nguyen C, Duque J, Woods S. Mobilization of malignant ascites with diuretics is dependent on ascitic fluid characteristics. Gastroenterology. 1992;**103**(4):1302-1306

[100] Sharma S, Walsh D. Management of symptomatic malignant ascites with diuretics: Two case reports and a review of the literature. Journal of Pain and Symptom Management. 1995;**10**(3):237-242. DOI: 10.1016/0885-3924(94)00129-9

[101] Chung M, Kozuch P. Treatment of malignant ascites. Current Treatment Options in Oncology. 2008;**9**(2-3):215-233. DOI: 10.1007/s11864-008-0068-y

[102] Wiest R, Schölmerich J. Diagnostik und Therapie des Aszites. Deutsches Ärzteblatt Heft. 2006;**28-29**:A1972-A1981

[103] Loggie BW, Perini M, Fleming RA, Russell GB, Geisinger K. Treatment and prevention of malignant ascites associated with disseminated intraperitoneal malignancies by aggressive combined-modality therapy. American Surgeon. 1997;**63**:137-143

[104] Kaufmann M, Schmid H, Raeth U, Grischke EM, Kempeni J, Schlick E, et al. Therapy of ascites with tumor necrosis factor in ovarian cancer. Geburtshilfe Frauenheilkd. 1990;**50**(9):678-682. DOI: 10.1055/s-2008-1026344

[105] Sartori S, Nielsen I, Tassinari D, Trevisani L, Abbasciano V, Malacarne P. Evaluation of a standardized protocol of intracavitary recombinant interferon α-2b in the palliative treatment of malignant peritoneal effusions. A prospective pilot study. Oncology. 2001;**61**(3):192-196. DOI: 55374

[106] Smith EM, Jayson GC. The current and future management of malignant ascites. Clinical Oncology: A Journal of the Royal College of Radiologists. 2003;**15**(2):59-72

[107] Faught W, Kirkpatrick JR, Krepart GV, Heywood MS, Lotocki RJ. Peritoneovenous shunt for palliation of gynecologic malignant ascites. Journal of American College of Surgery. 1995;**180**(4):472-474

[108] Adam R, Adam Y. Malignant ascites: Past, present and future. Journal of American College of Surgery. 2004;**198**(6):999-1011. DOI: 10.1016/j.jamcollsurg.2004.01.035

[109] Kobold S, Hegewisch-Becker S, Oechsle K, Jordan K, Bokemeyer C, Atanackovic D. Intraperitoneal VEGF inhibition using Bevacizumab: A potential approach for the symptomatic treatment of malignant ascites? Oncologist. 2009;**14**(12):1242-1251. DOI: 10.1634/theoncologist.2009-0109

[110] Ferrara N, Hillan KJ, Novotny W. Bevacizumab (Avastin), a humanized anti-VEGF monoclonal antibody for cancer therapy. Biochemical and Biophysical Research Communication. 2005;**333**(2):328-335. DOI: 10.1016/j.bbrc.2005.05.132

[111] NC Institute. FDA Approval for Bevacizumab. 2016

[112] Jayson GC, Kerbel R, Ellis LM, Harris AL. Antiangiogenic therapy in oncology: Current status and future directions. Lancet. 2016;**388**:518-529. DOI: 10.1016/S0140-6736(15)010 88-0

[113] Pujade-Lauraine E, Hilpert F, Weber B, Reuss A, Poveda A, Kristensen G, et al. Bevacizumab combined with chemotherapy for platinum-resistant recurrent ovarian cancer: The AURELIA open-label randomized phase III trial. Journal of Clinical Oncology. 2014;**32**:1302-1308. DOI: 10.1200/JCO.2013.51.4489

[114] USFaD Administration. Drugs FDA: FDA Approved Drug Products, AVASTIN (BEVACIZUMAB). 2016

[115] Wimberger P, Gilet H, Gonschior AK, Heiss MM, Moehler M, Oskay-Oezcelik G, et al. Deterioration in quality of life (QoL) in patients with malignant ascites: results from a phase II/III study comparing paracentesis plus catumaxomab with paracentesis alone. Annals of Oncology. 2012;**23**(8):1979-1985. DOI: 10.1093/annonc/mds178

[116] Tangkijvanich P, Tresukosol D, Sampatanukul P, Sakdikul S, Voravud N, Mahachai V, et al. Telomerase assay for differentiating between malignancy-related and nonmalignant ascites. Clinical Cancer Research. 1999;**5**(9):2470-2475

[117] Cheung DK, Raaf JH. Selection of patients with malignant ascites for a peritoneovenous shunt. Cancer. 1982;**50**(6):1204-1209

Section 2

Treatment, Complications and Prognosis

Chapter 5

Ascites: Treatment, Complications, and Prognosis

Patricia Huelin, Jose Ignacio Fortea,
Javier Crespo and Emilio Fábrega

Additional information is available at the end of the chapter

http://dx.doi.org/10.5772/intechopen.70384

Abstract

Ascites is the most common complication in patients with cirrhosis. It can lead to several life-threatening complications resulting in a poor long-term survival outcome. Ascites is due to the loss of compensatory mechanism to maintain effective arterial blood volume secondary to splanchnic arterial vasodilatation in the progression of liver disease and portal hypertension. Refractory ascites, spontaneous bacterial peritonitis (SBP), hyponatremia, and hepatorenal syndrome (HRS) are complications that can occur with ascites, all of them leading to a worse quality of life and short-term mortality. When complication appears, liver transplantation as a definitive and curative treatment should be considered. Other common therapeutical approaches to control ascites such as diet, sodium restriction, or the use of diuretics are needed to avoid these complications, although some patients will require further treatments when ascites becomes refractory to standard treatment. This chapter will review the complex treatment of ascites, and its related complications.

Keywords: ascites, hepatorenal syndrome, hyponatremia, portal hypertension, spontaneous bacterial peritonitis

1. Introduction

Decompensated cirrhosis is the end stage of chronic liver disease of any etiology. It has a wide range of different clinical manifestations that are secondary to portal hypertension and/or liver insufficiency. Ascites is the most frequent decompensation, and it is usually the first manifestation of the disease in the majority of the patients [1]. Ascites is the accumulation of liquid inside of the peritoneal cavity, and it is developed in 60% of patients with compensated cirrhosis within 10 years during the natural course of their liver disease [1]. Hippocrates of Kos described ascites a long time ago (ca. 460–ca. 310 BC), and its treatment with large paracentesis was already performed since the ancient Greek physicians. It is still a very common problem in patients with liver cirrhosis, malignancy, or cardiovascular disease today. As in Western Europe and the United States of America, liver cirrhosis is the main cause of ascites (75–85%), and we will focus on this disease [2, 3].

The development of ascites is the consequence of the action of several complex mechanisms secondary to severe portal hypertension (i.e., hepatic venous pressure gradient (HVPG) >12 mm Hg) giving place to an impairment of hepatic, circulatory, and renal function. Portal hypertension induces the activation of the endogenous vasoactive systems, which prevent the renal excretion of an adequate amount of sodium, leading to a positive sodium balance [4]. Large evidence suggests that renal sodium retention in patients with cirrhosis is secondary to arterial splanchnic vasodilation. This causes a decrease in effective arterial blood volume with activation of arterial and cardiopulmonary volume receptors, and homeostatic activation of vasoconstrictor and sodium retaining systems (i.e., renin-angiotensin-aldosterone, vasopressin, and the sympathetic nervous systems). Renal sodium retention leads to expansion of the extracellular fluid volume and increases intestinal capillary pressure. The latter is further increased due to both portal hypertension and splanchnic arterial vasodilatation, which also disrupts the intestinal capillary permeability, and thereby contributes to the accumulation of fluid in the abdominal cavity [5]. In addition, certain polymorphisms of the aquaporin-1 gene could predispose to water retention [6].

The development of ascites is associated with a poor prognosis and impaired quality of life in patients with cirrhosis [7]. The probability of survival at 1 and 5 years after decompensation by ascites is about 50 and 20%, respectively [8]. Because of the poor survival, and other complications that will be explained later, patients with ascites should generally be considered for referral for liver transplantation [3].

2. Evaluation and initial investigations

2.1. History and physical examination

The first step in the management of every patient with a new-onset ascites is to reveal its underlying cause. A thorough history and physical examination will help narrow the differential diagnosis and reveal factors that might have been implicated in the development of ascites (e.g., nonsteroidal anti-inflammatory drugs (NSAIDs)). Risk factors for liver disease such as alcohol abuse, metabolic syndrome, or family history of hemochromatosis should be sought. Patients should also be questioned about past history of cancer, heart failure, renal disease, or tuberculosis as they may all be responsible for the development of ascites [3].

The main complaint of patients with ascites is an increase in abdominal girth, often accompanied by lower-extremity edema. Other common manifestations include dyspnea due to increasing abdominal distension and/or accompanying pleural effusions, abdominal pain, anorexia, nausea, and fatigue [9]. The accuracy of the physical examination to detect ascites is highly dependent on the amount of ascites and on the physical constitution of the patient. Accordingly, patients must have approximately 1500 mL of fluid for ascites to be detected reliably by physical examination and the presence of obesity greatly reduces its diagnostic accuracy [3]. Several signs support the presence of ascites such as the shifting dullness, fluid wave, and puddle signs. The former has 83% sensitivity and 56% specificity in detecting ascites. It is also less cumbersome and performs better than the latter two [3, 10]. The clinician should also look for other physical signs that suggest the presence of a liver disease (e.g., spider angiomas, Dupuytren contracture, palmar erythema, gynecomastia, parotid gland enlargement, or testicular atrophy) or an extra-hepatic disease (e.g. jugular venous distension related to heart failure) as the cause of ascites.

2.2. Initial investigations

The essential investigations that should follow the anamnesis and physical examination to confirm the cause of ascites include an abdominal ultrasound (to screen for morphologic evidence of cirrhosis and portal hypertension, tumors, portal vein thrombosis, and hepatic vein thrombosis), laboratory assessment of liver function, renal function, serum and urine electrolytes, and abdominal paracentesis. The latter is compulsory in order to confirm the cause of the ascites and to rule out complications such as spontaneous bacterial peritonitis (SBP). Thus, it should always be performed in a new episode of ascites grades 2 or 3, in patients hospitalized for any complication of the disease or because of worsening of ascites [2, 11]. It is a safe procedure, even in patients with prolonged prothrombin time and low platelets. Indeed, the policy of some physicians to give blood products (fresh frozen plasma and/or platelets) routinely in these patients is not data-supported [3]. Growing evidence from the last two decades has demonstrated that most patients with liver cirrhosis remain in a tenous but balanced state of hemostasis [12]. Accordingly, in a study of 1100 large volume paracentesis, there were no hemorrhagic complications despite no prophylactic correction of platelet counts as low as 19,000 cells/mm^3 (54% < 50,000) and of prolonged international normalized ratios for prothrombin time as high as 8.7 (75% > 1.5 and 26.5% > 2.0) [13]. The most common site for paracentesis is the left lower quadrant of the abdominal wall (3 cm cephalad and 3 cm medial to the anterior superior iliac spine), as in this location the wall is thinner and with a larger pool of fluid than the midline. Visible collateral must be avoided, and in patients with obesity or loculated ascites, an ecoguided paracentesis is commonly needed [3].

The analysis of the ascitic fluid includes cell count and differential, culture, biochemical analysis, and cytology. Current guidelines recommend to routinely perform only cell count and differential, ascitic fluid protein and albumin, and note the gross appearance of the fluid (i.e., water-clear, bilious, purulent, bloody, or chylous) [2, 3]. The former enables to discard SBP or suspect the presence of other type of infection (e.g., high lymphocyte count in patients with tuberculosis). Albumin measurement on the same day in serum and ascitic fluid allows the calculation of the serum-ascites albumin gradient (SAAG), which properly differentiates ascites due to portal hypertension from ascites due to other causes. If the SAAG is greater than or equal to 1.1 g/dL, ascites is ascribed to portal hypertension with an approximate 97% accuracy [14]. Importantly, SAAG accuracy is not influenced by fluid infusion and diuretic use and also remains greater or equal to 1.1 g/dL in patients with both portal hypertension and a second cause for ascites formation [3]. Measurement of SAAG is, therefore, of utmost importance in patients with new-onset ascites, but its repeated measurement is usually not needed in other scenarios (e.g., worsening or refractory ascites) [3]. **Table 1** shows the etiological classification of ascites according to the SAAG value. Further ascitic testing should be done depending on clinical judgment [3]. In patients in whom a peritoneal carcinomatosis is suspected, an ascitic fluid cytology must be performed, as it has a sensitivity as high as 96.7% if three samples from different paracentesis procedures are analyzed [15]. Bacterial culture is mandatory if infection is suspected. Cultures should be done in aerobic and anaerobic blood cultures inoculated (10 mL) at the bedside to increase their profitability (80% by this method). The utility of lactate

SAAG	Diseases	Diagnosis
≥1.1	*Liver cirrhosis*	Compatible image test and biopsy, known etiology of liver disease, HVPG > 10 mm Hg, liver stiffness >15 Kpa, proteins in ascites <2.5 g/L
	Budd-Chiari syndrome	Imaging test, proteins in ascites >2.5 g/L
	Sinusoidal obstruction syndrome	Appropriate clinical context (e.g. hemotopoietic stem cell transplantation), proteins in ascites >2.5 g/L
	Portal thrombosis	Imaging test, usually associated with a clinical trigger such as variceal bleeding
	Right heart failure	Right heart failure confirmed by echocardiogram, serum BNP >364 pg/mL, dilated suprahepatic veins, proteins in ascites >2.5 g/L
	Acute liver failure	Appropriate clinical context
	Massive liver metastases	Imaging test, proteins in ascites <2.5 g/L
	Myxedema	Clinical and laboratory findings of severe hypothyroidism
	*"Mixed" ascites**	Imaging or other test according to clinical suspicion
<1.1	*Peritoneal carcinomatosis*	Positive citology, proteins in ascites >2.5 g/L, WBC >500 with PMNs<250, image test to find primary tumor (most frequent ovarian, gastric, and pancreatic origin)
	Peritoneal tuberculosis	WBC > 500 with PMNs<250 and predominance of lymphocytes, proteins in ascites >2.5 g/L, ADA >40 UI/L, positive culture or PCR, peritoneal biopsy
	Pancreatic ascitis	Ascitic amylase level usually >2000 UI/L, protein concentration in ascites variable, but normally >2.5 g/L, PMN > 250, imaging test to diagnose the underlying disease
	Bilious ascites	Elevated ascitic bilirubin levels and higher than serum, imaging test to diagnose the underlying disease
	Chylous ascites	Ascitic triglyceride level >110–200 mg/dL or higher than serum, imaging test to diagnose the underlying disease
	Nephrotic syndrome	Appropriate clinical context, proteins in ascites <2.5 g/L
	Protein-losing enteropathy	Diarrhea and other clinical symptoms due to the underlying disease, proteins in ascites <2.5 g/L
	Serositis related to connective tissue diseases	Rare manifestación of systemic lupus erythematosus, polyarteritis nodosa and Schölein-Henoch purpura. Appropriate clinical context
	Intestinal ischemia or obstruction	Imaging test

*Patients with cirrhosis and other cause (one or more) of ascites formation. Abbreviations: SAAG: serum-ascites albumin gradient; HVPG: hepatic venous pressure gradient; WCC: white blood cell; PMN: polymorphonuclear leukocyte; ADA: adenosine deaminase; PCR: polymerase chain reaction.

Table 1. Etiological classification of ascites according to the serum-ascites albumin gradient value.

dehydrogenase and glucose determination in ascitic fluid to assist in differentiating spontaneous from secondary bacterial peritonitis is supported by limited data and the European Association for the Study of the Liver (EASL) does not recommend its performance [2]. On the contrary, an ascitic fluid carcinoembryonic antigen >5 ng/mL or ascitic fluid alkaline phosphatase >240 units/L has been shown to be accurate in detecting gut perforation into ascitic fluid [16]. Other tests, such as amylase, triglycerides, and polymerase chain reaction (PCR) and culture for mycobacteria should be done only when there is a clinical suspicion of pancreatic disease, chylous ascites, and tuberculosis, respectively. Finally, it is worth mentioning that serum cancer antigen 125 levels are increased in patients with ascites of any cause. Therefore, its measurement is not recommended to guide the differential diagnosis [3].

3. Treatment of ascites

Current guidelines follow the classification of ascites from the International Ascites Club, which divides patients into three groups on the basis of a quantitative criterion. Each group is also linked to a specific treatment strategy (see **Table 2**) [3, 17]. Accordingly, only patients with ascites grade 2 or more should be treated, and they can be treated as outpatients unless they have other complications [2]. The aim of the treatment of ascites is to induce negative sodium balance by reducing sodium intake and increasing sodium excretion by the administration of diuretics.

3.1. Sodium restriction

In approximately 10–20% of patients with cirrhosis and ascites, we can obtain a negative sodium balance only by reducing dietary sodium intake, particularly in those presenting with their first episode of ascites [18]. No predictive factors of response to low sodium diet have been detected. Although the level of dietary restriction should be applied according to the baseline urinary sodium excretion, a moderate restriction of salt intake is generally recommended (intake of sodium of 80–120 mmol/day, which corresponds to 4.6–6.9 g of salt/day). This is generally equivalent to a no-added salt diet with avoidance of preprepared meals. A more severe reduction in dietary sodium content is considered unnecessary and even

Severity and definition	Treatment and strategy
Grade 1 or mild Diagnosed exclusively by ultrasonography.	No treatment is necessary.
Grade 2 or moderate Clinically evident.	Dietary sodium restriction and diuretics. (first spironolactone 50–100 mg/day to reach weight loss: 300–500 mg/day, if needed, add furosemide 20–40 mg/day and increase both every 7 days up to 400 and 160 mg/day, respectively)
Grade 3 or large Clinically evident or tense.	Large-volume paracentesis plus albumin 8 g/L of ascites removed in first place and later dietary sodium restriction (90 mmol/day) and diuretics.

Table 2. Ascites classification and treatment [17].

potentially deleterious since it may impair nutritional status [2, 3]. Fluid restriction is not necessary unless patients have hypovolemic hyponatremia (serum sodium <130 mEq/L together with ascites and/or edema). Fluid loss and weight change are directly related to sodium balance in these patients. It is sodium restriction, not fluid restriction, which results in weight loss, as fluid follows sodium passively [2].

3.2. Diuretics

Evidence demonstrates that renal sodium retention is mainly due to increased proximal as well as distal tubular sodium reabsorption rather than due to a decrease of filtered sodium load [2, 19]. The increased reabsorption of sodium along the distal tubule is mostly related to hyperaldosteronism. As previously mentioned, patients with ascites grade 2 require diuretic treatment if there is no contraindication. The goal of treatment is to achieve an average weight loss of no more than 500 g/day in patients without peripheral edema and no more than 800–1000 g/day in those with peripheral edema.

The efficacy of diuretic therapy in the control of ascites is approximately 90% in patients without renal dysfunction [2, 19]. The diuretics most frequently used are aldosterone antagonists, mainly spironolactone, which selectively antagonizes the sodium-retaining effects of aldosterone in the renal collecting tubules, and loop diuretics, especially furosemide, that inhibit the Na + –K + –2Cl – cotransporter in the loop of Henle. It has been extensively debated whether both types of diuretics should be combined from the beginning or use aldosterone antagonists in a stepwise increase every 7 days with furosemide added only in patients not responding to high doses of aldosterone antagonists. It can be concluded that a diuretic regime based on the combination of aldosterone antagonists and furosemide is the most adequate approach for patients with recurrent ascites but not for patients with a first episode of ascites. These latter patients respond well to spironolactone 50–100 mg/day [2]. Those with recurrent episodes of ascites or peripheral edema should receive a combination of spironolactone 100 mg/day with furosemide 40 mg/day [2, 19]. If there is no response, adherence to a low sodium-diet and diuretic treatment should be confirmed through a good anamnesis and a 24-hour urine sodium excretion measurement. An ascites that is not controlled despite a natriuresis greater than 80–110 mmol/day suggests a non-adherence to a low-sodium diet [3]. Given that full-day collections are cumbersome, the measurement of urine creatinine helps determine if the collection of the 24-hour specimen has been complete. Men with cirrhosis should excrete more than 15 mg of creatinine/kg of body weight per day, and women should excrete more than 10 mg/kg/day. Less creatinine is indicative of an incomplete collection [3]. A random "spot" urine sample is also useful to assess natriuresis and is the preferable test to adjust diuretic treatment in certain scenarios such as the emergency unit. A sodium concentration that is greater than the potassium concentration correlates well with a 24-hour sodium excretion. When the urine sodium/potassium ratio is >1, the patient should be responding to the treatment. The higher the ratio, the greater the urine sodium excretion [20]. In compliant patients with poorly controlled ascites, diuretics may then be increased every 7 days by doubling doses (1:1 ratio) to a maximal dose of spironolactone (400 mg/day) and a maximal dose of furosemide (160 mg/day). Unfortunately, diuretics can also have side effects and cause fluid and electrolytes balance disturbances such as hyponatremia, dehydration, renal impairment, hyperkalemia, or hypokalemia and subsequently, hepatic encephalopathy. For all these reasons, patients should be closely followed after the onset of diuretic treatment. Thus, a clinical evaluation and measurements of serum and urine electrolytes must be performed within the first 2 weeks after starting or modifying their dose. When any of the abovementioned side effects appear, diuretics should be stopped or their dose reduced. A particular side effect of spironolactone is tender gynecomastia and muscle cramps in some patients. Amiloride, a diuretic acting in the collecting duct, is less effective than aldosterone antagonists and should be used only in those patients who develop severe side effects with aldosterone antagonists [2].

3.3. Other general measures

Treatment of the underlying disease whenever possible is of great importance as dramatic responses have been described after alcohol abstinence, antiviral, and immunosuppressive therapies in patients with alcoholic, viral and autoimmune liver diseases, respectively [3]. Nutritional therapy can ameliorate nutritional status in cirrhotic patients, reduce infection rates, and decrease perioperative morbidity [11]. Some drugs must be avoided or use with caution in patients with ascites such as NSAID due to the high risk of developing further sodium retention, hyponatremia, and renal failure. In a recent case control study, 37% of the NSAIDs-associated acute kidney injury (AKI) cases were severe and persistent with a very poor short-term outcome [21]. Interestingly, Metamizol use was more common in patients with persistent AKI than in those with transient AKI, and therefore, this drug should also be used with caution. Likewise, angiotensin converting enzyme inhibitors, angiotensin II antagonists, or a1-adrenergic receptor blockers should generally not be used in patients with ascites because of increased risk of renal impairment [2]. Bed rest was previously recommended on the basis that the upright posture could aggravate the already elevated plasma renin levels of patients with liver cirrhosis and ascites. However, it is no longer advocated as there is insufficient evidence to support its use as part of ascites treatment [2]. There is an ongoing debate about the use of nonselective betablockers in patients with refractory ascites. The current guidelines from the American Association for the Study of Liver Diseases recommend to avoid high doses of these drugs (over 160 mg/day of propranolol or over 80 mg/day of nadolol), and in patients with concomitant severe circulatory dysfunction [i.e., systolic blood pressure <90 mm Hg, serum sodium <130 mEq/L, or hepatorenal syndrome (HRS)], their dose should be decreased or the drug temporarily held [22]. Finally, in unblinded randomized clinical trials (RCTs), the long-term albumin infusion (25 g weekly for one year and 25 g every two weeks thereafter) improved survival in patients with new onset ascites [23]. However, further studies are needed before this treatment can be advocated [3].

4. Complications, prognosis, and treatment

Despite the fact that patients with ascites constitute a heterogeneous population with different prognosis depending on the degree of liver insufficiency and circulatory dysfunction, the development of ascites is an ominous sign. The probability of survival at one and five years after the diagnosis of ascites is approximately 50 and 20%, respectively, and long-term survival of more than 10 years is very rare [8]. In addition, mortality rises up to 80% within 6–12 months in patients who also develop kidney failure [1]. Patients with cirrhosis and ascites are also at high risk for other life-threatening complications of liver disease, including refractory ascites, SBP, respiratory distress, worsening of nutritional status, hyponatremia, or HRS. Accordingly, current guidelines recommend that every patient with ascites should be generally considered for referral for liver transplantation, especially when quality of life is impaired due to refractory ascites, or in the presence of SBE and HRS [2, 3]. Since 2002, the model of end-stage liver disease (MELD) score is used for patient priority in liver transplantation. However, MELD does not reflect the impact of some complications (the so-called Exceptions to MELD score) such as refractory ascites. Indeed, in some patients with this complication the latter score does not accurately reflect their poor prognosis (median survival is approximately 6 months) and their prioritization in the list should be assessed [24].

4.1. Refractory ascites

A nonnegligible number of patients with ascites (10%) develop refractory ascites due to severe sodium retention that cannot be mobilized pharmacologically either because there is no response to high diuretic dose (resistant ascites) or because side effects appear with the use of diuretics (intractable ascites). The term "recurrent ascites" defines an ascites that requires more than three admissions per year because of reaccumulation of ascites [25]. In these patients other therapeutical approaches must be used.

4.1.1. Large volume paracentesis (LVP)

Current guidelines recommend LVP as the first-line treatment in patients with refractory ascites, unless it is loculated [2, 3]. In order to minimize the number of paracentesis (LVP is usually performed every 2–4 weeks), total paracentesis is preferred and diuretic therapy can be maintained if the urine sodium is >30 mmol/day. It is a safe procedure with a complicate rate similar to diagnostic paracentesis, and it can be performed in the outpatient setting [2, 3]. LVP is defined as a volume above 5 L. Although Kao et al. arbitrarily selected this threshold in 1985 based upon the volume required to "adequately decompress the distended abdomen," the intra-individual neurohormonal changes induced by the removal of different ascitic volumes have not been examined [26, 27]. These neurohormonal changes reflect the physiopathological background of the main complication of LP, i.e., postparacentesis circulatory dysfunction (PPCD). Indeed, the removal of large volumes of ascites fluid can further decline the effective circulating volume by causing a significant drop in peripheral vascular resistance by mechanisms not fully elucidated. This hemodynamic derangement is demonstrated by a pronounced reactivation of renin-angiotensin-aldosterone and sympathetic nervous systems that can persist for months. An increase in plasma renin activity of 50% or greater is usually used to define PPCD [27, 28]. Although frequently asymptomatic, PPCD has been associated with significant detrimental effects such as re-accumulation of ascites, development of HRS and dilutional hyponatremia, and shortened survival [2]. It was first demonstrated in the 1980s that adjunctive albumin infusion can prevent PPCD occurrence and since the early 1990s, less costly alternatives to albumin have been sought, such as artificial colloid volume expanders and vasoconstrictors [28]. Despite initial uncertain results, a meta-analysis of

17 trials with a total 1225 patients demonstrated that albumin infusion after LVP is more effective than other plasma expanders (i.e., hypertonic saline, hydroxyethyl starch, and dextran-70, polygeline) for the prevention of PPCD and showed a trend to increased survival. The rate of PPCD was 73% after paracentesis without any re-expansion, 38% when combined with an infusion of dextran or gelatin solutions and only 15–17% when taps were combined with albumin administration. Doses of albumin infusion ranged between 5 and 10 g of albumin per liter of fluid removed [28]. Current guidelines recommend 8 g/L as this has been the dose most commonly used [2, 3]. It is usually administered during or after the paracentesis. Whether lower doses could be used is currently debated as one study comparing doses of 4 vs. 8 g/L showed similar efficacy in preventing PPCD and renal impairment [29]. When less than 5 L of ascites are removed, artificial plasma expanders, saline, and albumin are equally effective [2]. The latter meta-analysis also compared albumin with vasoconstrictors (i.e., midodrine, norepinephrine, and terlipressin). The results were more variable in this subgroup (OR from 0.30 to 5.54) due to the small size of the five included trials and therefore, no definitive conclusions can be made [28]. Further studies that target survival as the primary end-point in patients with truly refractory ascites are needed to fully demonstrate whether albumin or vasoconstrictors can improve survival.

4.1.2. Transjugular intrahepatic portosystemic shunt (TIPS)

Another treatment option for patients with refractory ascites is transjugular intrahepatic portosystemic shunt (TIPS). It is a procedure in which an intrahepatic stent is inserted between the hepatic and portal veins with intent for portal decompression to avoid the recurrence of ascites [30]. The optimal portal pressure gradient (PPG) that needs to be obtained to adequately control ascites is not clear, but might be lower than the well-validated 12 mm Hg threshold for the prevention of rebleeding from esophageal varices [30]. Most of randomized clinical trials (RCTs) aimed to reduce PPG below 12 mm Hg by dilating 10-mm diameter stents to 6–8 mm with subsequent calibration up to 10 mm, depending on post-PPG and clinical response [31–34]. By this approach, marked reductions in PPG are avoided, which may be associated with an increased risk of hepatic encephalopathy and liver failure. Until today, seven RCT [31–37] and six meta-analysis [38–43] have assessed the efficacy and safety of TIPS in patients with refractory and recurrent ascites. They have consistently demonstrated that TIPS is effective in the management of this complication, but is associated with higher risk of hepatic encephalopathy compared to LVP. Thus, about 64% (range of 38–84%) had their ascites controlled (although its resolution was slow and most patients required continued administration of diuretics and salt restriction), and hepatic encephalopathy occurred in approximately 51% of patients (39% severe) treated with TIPS. This latter complication is known to increase the rate of mortality and hospitalization and to significantly affect the quality of life [30]. TIPS dysfunction due to pseudointimal hyperplasia within the parenchymal tract or within the outflow hepatic vein was another major drawback in these studies. Indeed, a significant proportion of patients (from 30 to 87%) needed TIPS revision due to malfunction. It must be emphasized that all, but one clinical trial [34], used bare stents instead of the politetrafluoroethylene-covered stents that are used today. These covered-stents have greatly improved shunt patency rates and have also reduced the incidence of hepatic encephalopathy after TIPS placement [30]. There is great controversy over the survival benefit of TIPS in refractory ascites. At the time current guidelines were published, studies had not convincingly proved that TIPS improved survival compared to repeated LVP, and consequently, it was left as a second-line therapy that had to be considered in patients with very frequent requirement of LVP or with loculated ascites [2, 3]. Among the five trials that had been published at that time, transplant-free survival was significantly improved in two (in one of them only in the multivariate analysis) [33, 36], decreased in one (probably due to technical disability) [35], and not affected in the other two [31, 37]. These discrepancies among studies were likely due to patient selection and data analysis biases. These RCTs excluded patients with advanced liver disease (as defined by serum bilirubin > 5–6 mg/dL, INR > 2, current or chronic HE > 2 by West-Heaven scale), and renal failure (as defined by serum creatinine >3 mg/dL) and thus, only 48% (median, 21–77%) of the screened patients could be included in the RCTs. Meta-analysis also contributed to this controversy. Four conventional meta-analysis did not show any benefit in survival [38–41], whereas a meta-analysis of individual patient data from four RCT showed a significant improvement in transplant-free survival at 1 and 2 years between TIPS and LVP (63 and 49% vs. 53 and 35%, $p = 0.035$) [42]. After the publication of the current guidelines, two RCT [32, 34] and another meta-analysis [43] have been published and concluded that TIPS is more effective in controlling ascites than repeated LVP and improved transplant-free survival in these patients. The RCT of Narahara et al. included 60 patients with refractory ascites treated with bare metal TIPS or LVP. The selection criteria were stricter than the previous RCT and included patients with better preserved renal and hepatic function [32]. The last RCT was recently published and included patients with recurrent ascites treated with covered-stents or LVP with inclusion criteria similar to the former RCT [34]. It can be concluded that pending further RCT with covered stents, TIPS can be recommended in patients with refractory ascites and preserved liver function (Child–Pugh score <13, MELD score <18, bilirubin <5 mg/dL, platelet count >75,000, serum sodium >130 mEq/L), aged <70, no previous episodes of hepatic encephalopathy, and neither central or large hepatocellular carcinoma nor cardiopulmonary disease [19]. In fact, some authors and scientific associations recommend TIPS as the primary therapy for refractory ascites [44–46].

4.1.3. Automated low flow pump system (Alfapump System)

The alfapump is a subcutaneous battery-operated pump to move ascites from the peritoneum to the urinary bladder. One catheter connects the pump to the peritoneal cavity, and another connects it to the urinary bladder. Every 5–10 min small volumes of ascites (generally 5–10 mL) are pumped into the urinary bladder, ranging the daily volume that can be removed between 500 mL and 2.5 L. In order to improve patient's comfort it is deactivated at night. The pump battery is charged via a charging device (Smart Charger, Sequana Medical AG, Zürich, Switzerland) that is placed over the area of the pump twice daily during no more than 20 min. It is at this time when pump function parameters (e.g., volumen transported, pressures in the bladder and abdominal cavity) are automatically transmitted to the charger. This information is forwarded to a central databank and communicated, if needed, to the treating physician, who can remotely program the system to the patient's needs or contact the patient because of possible technical issues. The current price of the device is 22,500 Euros [47].

The alfapump was conceived as an alternative treatment for refractory ascites, especially in those patients who are not candidates for TIPS [47, 48]. This system also requires a good selection process, in which issues such as compliance of the patient, nutritional status, previous abdominal surgery, urinary outlet obstruction, or local skin infections should be carefully evaluated before its implantation [47]. An initial multicenter, prospective, uncontrolled study (PIONEER) evaluated its safety and efficacy in 40 patients over a period of 6 months. It showed that the pump removed 90% of the ascites and reduced the median number of LVP, but with a significant rate of complications mainly due to infections and catheter dislodgement [49]. However, the number of complications was reduced along the study after including some changes recommended by the data safety monitoring board (i.e., antibiotic prophylaxis with norfloxacin, strict avoidance of NSAID, and the intravenous administration of albumin if ascites was aspired during the surgical intervention) [47]. A recent RCT compared the safety and efficacy of the alfapump system in comparison with LVP in 58 cirrhotic patients with refractory ascites over a 6-month period [48]. The alfapump was more effective reducing and, in many cases, eliminating (more than 50%) the need for paracentesis. It also improved the quality of life and nutritional status of the patients. Survival was similar in both groups, despite the occurrence of more adverse events (96.3 vs. 77.4%, $p = 0.057$), which were also more frequently severe (85.2% vs. 45.2%, $p = 0.002$) in the group treated with alfapump. Adverse events consisted predominantly of AKI in the immediate post-operative period, and re-intervention for pump-related issues. Device deficiencies accounted for seven re-interventions, which are an improvement compared to the results of the PIONEER study and may reflect the continual technological improvements to the alfapump system since commercialization in 2011. After the postoperative period (>7 days), the incidence of AKI and hyponatremia was similar in both groups, but more of these events required hospitalization in the alfapump group. The underlying mechanism for this renal dysfunction and hyponatremia remains unclear. In a recent prospective study that included ten patients with refractory ascites treated with the alfapump system, a marked activation of endogenous vasoconstrictor systems and impairment of kidney function after the device insertion was observed. This finding led the authors to hypothesize that treatment with alfapump might impair effective arterial blood volume mimicking a postparacentesis circulatory dysfunction syndrome and suggested a potential role of albumin in counteracting these effects [50]. Supporting this hypothesis, the authors of the RCT observed an increase in plasma renin activity at 3 months. Finally, total median cost (including implantation procedure and device, scheduled visits, lab test, medications and treatment of adverse events) was significantly higher in the alfapump group (£36970 vs. £12660, $p < 0.0001$). The difference was primarily due to the statistically higher cost of implantation procedure and adverse effects [48]. It can be concluded that further refinements in patient selection, patient care algorithms (including regular albumin administration), and modifications in device design are needed before the alfapump can become a truly alternative treatment for patients with refractory ascites.

4.1.4. Vaptans

Vaptans are V2 vasopressin receptor antagonists acting on the kidney and promoting solute-free water diuresis. In patients with cirrhosis, they have been studied in the setting of dilutional hyponatremia (see below section 6) and ascites. In patients with both uncomplicated and refractory ascites, satavaptan did not have a clinical benefit in controlling ascites and even increased mortality, which was related with known complications of liver cirrhosis [51, 52]. Consequently, the drug was withdrawn from development. Tolvaptan has also been used in patients with liver cirrhosis and refractory ascites. Most of the data come from observational studies in which tolvaptan seemed to improve control of ascites [53–57]. Two RCT also showed that tolvaptan was more effective than placebo for the treatment of ascites-related clinical symptoms. However, in both trials, the drug was given for only 7 days and the follow-up period was no longer than 3 weeks [58, 59]. Both issues are of great concern, given that its efficacy is lost after the discontinuation of the drug [60] and that a black-box warning by the Food and Drug Administration determined that tolvaptan should not be used for longer than 30 days, and limited its use in patients with underlying liver disease. The latter warning came from an increased risk of liver injury in a recent large clinical trial evaluating tolvaptan for a new use in patients with autosomal dominant polycystic kidney disease [61]. Therefore, the use of vaptans in cirrhotic patients with uncomplicated or refractory ascites cannot be recommended at present and required further RCT with a longer follow-up [3, 11].

4.1.5. Vasoconstrictors

Since arterial splanchnic vasodilation plays a major role in the pathogenesis of ascites formation, the use of vasoconstrictors has been evaluated in the treatment of patients with refractory or recurrent ascites. In two preliminary studies both the acute and 7-day administration of Midodrine, an alfa-1-adrenergic agonist, in nonazotemic cirrhotic patients with ascites improved systemic hemodynamics and sodium excretion [62, 63]. Similarly, in another study, the addition of midodrine corrected the deleterious effects on renal function of octreotide and improved systemic hemodynamics [64]. The first study evaluating its effect on patients with refractory or recurrent ascites was a RCT in which 40 patients were randomized to oral midodrine (7.5 mg every 8 h) plus standard medical therapy (sodium restriction plus diuretics) or to standard medical therapy alone. Midodrine significantly improved systemic hemodynamics without significant complications and was superior for the control of ascites at 3 months, but not at 1 and 6 months after therapy. Moreover, the mortality rate in the standard medical therapy group was significantly higher than that in the midodrine group ($p < 0.046$) [65]. A recent pilot study evaluated the efficacy and safety of midodrine in combination with tolvaptan in 50 cirrhotic patients with refractory or recurrent ascites. Their combination controlled ascites significantly better than standard diuretic treatment alone and more rapidly than midodrine alone [66].

Clonidine, a centrally acting α2-agonist and sympatholytic agent, has also been evaluated as an adjunct treatment in patients with cirrhosis and refractory ascites. In two pilot studies, its addition to spironolactone increased natriuresis and body weight loss more efficiently than spironolactone alone in patients with cirrhosis and ascites and activated sympathetic nervous system [67, 68]. Years later, the same group performed a first RCT that included patients with cirrhosis, ascites, and a plasma norepinephrine level of >300 pg/mL. Oral clonidine (0.075 mg b.i.d.) led to an earlier duretic response and was associated with fewer diuretic requirements and complications [69]. A later RCT using the same dose of clonidine for 3 months evaluated its efficacy in 270 patients with refractory ascites. The response rate to the association of clonidine and diuretics was 55–60%. The highest efficacy was obtained in patients who had high serum levels of norepinephine and the presence of two specific polymorphisms of the G-protein and α2-adrenergic receptor gene [70]. The efficacy of the combination of clonidine and midrodine was evaluated in a RCT that included 60 patients with refractory and recurrent ascites. Their combination controlled ascites significantly better than standard diuretic treatment alone over a 1-month period, but was not superior to midodrine or clonidine alone [71].

Finally, there is very limited data available with terlipressin. In a small RCT that included 15 patients with nonrefractory ascites and 8 with refractory ascites without HRS, 2 mg of intravenous terlipressin improved renal function and natriuresis in both types of ascites. However, a clinical effect on weight or abdominal girth was not recorded [72]. In a prospective study in which 26 patients with refractory ascites without HRS were treated with maximum diuretic treatment plus albumin and terlipressin, complete and partial response were observed in 62 and 23% of the patients, respectively [73].

With the available evidence, the American Association for the Study of Liver Diseases recommends that the use of oral midodrine should be considered in patients with refractory ascites [3]. On the other hand, the European Association for the Study of the Liver considers that larger RCT with longer follow-up are needed before these drugs can be routinely recommended in the management of these patients [2]. The authors of this chapter are in agreement with this last recommendation.

Figure 1 depicts the pathophysiological rationale for the treatment of patients with ascites and other related complications.

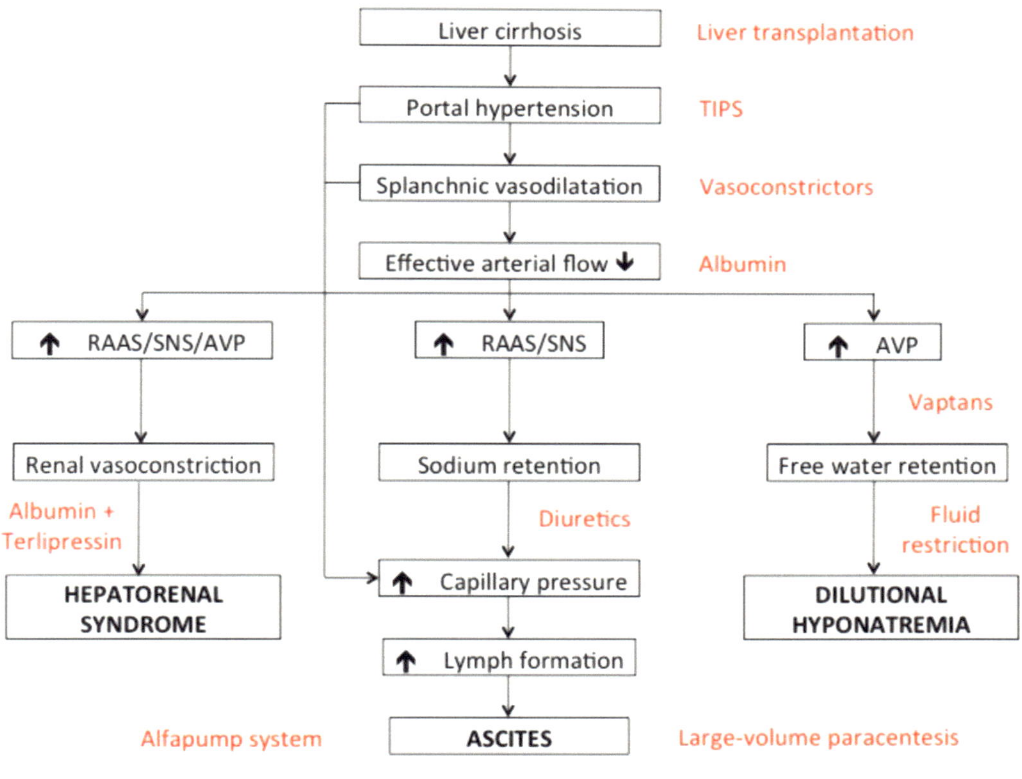

Figure 1. Physiopathology and treatment of patients with ascites and other related complications. Splanchnic vasodilatation driven by portal hypertension leads to an arterial underfilling that is counteracted by the activation of antinatriuretic and vasoconstrictor factors (RAAS, SNS, and AVP) that may lead to development of ascites, dilutional hyponatremia, and hepatorenal syndrome. Current therapies act at different levels of this pathophysiological cascade. Abbreviations: TIPS: transjugular intrahepatic portosystemic shunt; RAAS: renin-angotensin-aldosterone system; sympathetic nervous system; AVP: arginine vasopressin.

5. Spontaneous bacterial peritonitis (SBP)

Compared to general population, patients with cirrhosis have an increased risk of developing bacterial infections and sepsis, for this reason, SBP has a remarkable importance. SBP is a common infection of ascitic fluid developed in patients in the absence of an intra-abdominal genesis of infection. SBP was described for the first-time long time ago, approximately in the 1970s by Harold Conn [74], who pointed out the high in-hospital mortality in patients with this complication. The mechanisms leading to SBP include bacterial translocation, the reduced gut motility giving place to intestinal bacterial overgrowth, altered structure, and function of the intestinal mucosal barrier, and shortage in local immune response systems [75]. Patients with cirrhosis and SBP frequently develop an exaggerated inflammatory response with a severe impairment in renal, cardiovascular, or other organs functions. This syndrome is called acute or chronic liver failure and implies a high rate of hospital mortality [76].

SBP is the most frequent bacterial infection in hospitalized patients with cirrhosis [77]. It occurs in approximately 15–30% of hospitalized patients. Approximately 70% of the episodes of SBP is present when patients are admitted to the hospital, and the rest, 30%, is acquired during hospitalization [78]. The clinical manifestations in patients with SBP are usually symptoms such as abdominal pain, diarrhea, fever, chills, and hepatic encephalopathy, but in approximately 25% of cases of SBP, there are no apparent symptoms. Subclinical manifestations could occur as, for example, deterioration in renal function without other cause or development of tense and refractory ascites in a patient previously responsive to diuretics.

The prognosis in patients with SBP is very poor. The mortality during hospitalization is still remarkably high (20–40%) and is due to other complications that could appear because of the advanced liver disease. The most determinant prognostic factor in patients with SBP is the development of HRS [79]. The development of type-1 HRS and the poor short-term prognosis in these patients mostly depends on the degree of liver and renal impairment at diagnosis of SBP. There are several related-factors to an increased risk of type 1 HRS in patients with SBP; serum bilirubin levels ≥4 mg/dL, serum creatinine levels ≥1 mg/dL, and BUN ≥30 mg/dL [80–83]. In addition, SBP may trigger severe life-threatening complications, as for example, renal impairment, gastrointestinal bleeding, and deterioration of hepatic insufficiency, which are responsible for the associated high mortality.

The importance of an early diagnosis and the use of an adequate treatment are crucial in the survival. As previously mentioned, its diagnosis requires a polymorphonuclear leukocyte count greater than 250 cells/mm^3 [2]. The most common organisms isolated in SBP are *Escherichia coli, Klebsiella pneumoniae,* and *Streptococcus pneumoniae* [19]. The organism responsible for the infection is isolated in 60–70% of the cases. The remaining cases without the isolation of the organism are considered to have a culture-negative SBP and are treated in the same way as those with a positive culture. In the diagnostic procedure of SBP, must be a differentiation between SBP and secondary peritonitis. Secondary peritonitis is defined because it follows a primary abdominal infection such as gallbladder infection, diverticulitis, or gut perforation. Patients' general conditions rapidly deteriorates in those with secondary peritonitis, for this reason, the diagnosis must be quick, and can be confirmed by a laboratory workup, showing at least two of the following conditions: low glucose concentration levels in ascitic fluid (<50 mg/mL), ascites lactate dehydrogenase higher than serum lactate dehydrogenase, and finally, ascites concentration of proteins >1.5 g/dL. Other typical characteristics in secondary peritonitis are positive cultures with different bacteria, very high count of neutrophils in blood and ascitic fluid. When these conditions appear, a CT scan is recommended to localize the source of the infection [84, 85].

Current guidelines recommend the onset of the empirical treatment immediately after the diagnosis of the infection, and it should be performed with broad-spectrum antibiotics such as a third-generation cephalosporin [2, 3]. Until the last 10 years, the use of third-generation cephalosporins has been shown to be highly effective in the treatment of SBP. Gram-negative bacteria (particularly enterobacteriaceae) were responsible for the majority of the episodes of SBP [86]. However, the etiology and epidemiology in patients with cirrhosis and SBP have changed in the last years, and the efficacy of the third-generation cephalosporins as well as that of alternative therapies such as amoxicillin-clavulanic or quinolones has decreased [78]. It has been speculated that prophylaxis with norfloxacin and invasive procedures could have caused these changes [87].

Patients with nosocomial SBP have a high incidence of multidrug resistant (MDR) bacteria and have a poor response to third-generation cephalosporin in up to 25–66% of cases [78, 88]. Patients with an ineffective first-line treatment for SBP have been associated with very poor survival [86]. A group of experts suggested in 2014 a modification of the current guidelines in patients with nosocomial SBP by using a broader-spectrum of antibiotics, but it was not until last year, when a randomized controlled trial of 32 patients in Padua compared different antibiotic treatment of nosocomial SBP. Patients were randomized to receive meropenem plus daptomycin vs. cetazidime. After 48 hours of treatment, a paracentesis was performed and if the neutrophil count of the ascitic fluid decreased less than 25% compared to pretreatment value, it was considered a treatment failure. The main outcome was the resolution of SBP after 7 days of treatment. The arm with the combination of meropenem plus daptomycin was markedly more effective than the arm of only the third-generation cephalosporin (87 vs. 25%, respectively) with a p value of <0.001. In the study, 90-day transplant-free survival was also evaluated without significantly different values between both arms of treatment, and the last important issue to be described of the study, in the multivariate analysis of 90-day transplant-free survival. The independent predictive factors or survival were ineffective response to first-line treatment (hazard ratio: 20.6; $p < 0.01$), development of AKI throughout the hospitalization (HR: 23.2; $p < 0.01$), and baseline mean arterial pressure (HR: 0.92; $p < 0.01$) [89].

Different broad-spectrum of antibiotics have been proposed, but carbapenems should be used in order to widely cover the spectrum of Gram-negative MDR bacteria. Regarding Gram-positive bacteria, linezolid, lipo, or glycopeptides should be used, but there are some concerns about the high risk of nephrotoxicity and the high rate of vancomycin-resistant enterococci in patients with cirrhosis and nosocomial infections treated with glycopeptides. Duration of therapy should be a minimum of 5–7 days. In patients who develop renal impairment, it is recommended to use intravenous albumin (1.5 g/kg at diagnosis, followed by 1 g/kg on day 3) along with ceftriaxone [90]. The SBP resolution rate ranges between 70 and 90%. Despite the resolution of the infection, patients recovering from an episode of SBP should be considered as potential candidates for liver transplantation.

In patients who have had one episode of SBP, the recurrence rate within 1 year is 70% [91]. Long-term norfloxacin administration (400 mg/day p.o) decreases the recurrence within the first year after SBP from 68% in the placebo group to 20% in the treated group. Therefore, with these results, all patients with a previous episode of SBP should be treated with norfloxacin indefinitely until liver transplantation, death, or resolution of ascites [90, 92].

Prevention of SBP should always be considered especially in high-risk patients, including those with acute gastrointestinal hemorrhage, low ascitic fluid protein concentration (<10–15 g/L), survivors of a previous episode of SBP, and advanced cirrhosis [2]. A RCT showed that the administration of primary prophylaxis with norfloxacin in patients with low protein ascites (<15 g/L), advanced liver disease (Child Pugh score ≥9, serum bilirubin ≥ 3 mg/dL), or deterioration of kidney function (serum creatinine ≥1.2 mg/dL or serum sodium <130 mEq/L) significantly reduce several complications such as 1 year probability of developing SBP (from 61 to 7%), HRS (from 41 to 28%), and improved 3-month survival (from 62 to 94%) [83]. In addition, Soriano et al. demonstrated that intestinal decontamination with norfloxacin was useful to prevent SBP in hospitalized patients with low ascitic fluid protein levels (23 vs. 0%) [91]. Although prophylaxis strategies are beneficial in several aspects, long-term administration of antibiotics leads to the emergence of MDR bacteria as previously explained. However, due to the problem of antibiotic resistance, clinical judgment must guide the use of antibiotic prophylaxis [93]. Rifaximin has been recently proposed as a possible alternative treatment in prophylaxis of SBP. A case control study published many years ago showed that rifaximin was beneficial in the prevention of SBP in patients with hepatic encephalopathy [94]. Since then two studies have compared the efficacy of rifaximin vs. conventional prophylaxis (i.e., norfloxacin) and have provided contradictory results. In a prospective study including patients with and without previous SBP, rifaximin did not lead to a reduction of SBP occurrence in hospitalized patients with advanced liver disease, despite a greater proportion of patients with previous SBP in the norfloxacin group (89 vs. 15%, $p < 0.001$) [95]. Conversely, in a RCT including 260 patients with ascites and a previous episode of SBP, rifaximin was more effective than norfloxacin in reducing the recurrence of SBP (3.9% vs. 14.1%; $p = 0.04$) and even improved survival (13.7% vs. 24.4%; $p = 0.044$) during an 18 month of follow-up [96].

6. Hyponatremia

Furthermore, ascites is very often complicated by a disability of solute-free water excretion. In this setting, the antinatriuretic pathway involves the oversecretion of arginine vasopressin (AVP) that enhances the function of the vasopressin 2 (V2) receptors in the renal distal collecting tubules, inhibiting solute-free water excretion [97]. In this scenario, the AVP production is increased, and there is a lack of clearance of AVP due to cirrhosis itself. In addition, V2 is excessively bound by AVP, triggering more free water retention in kidney tubules by the creation of more aquaporin-2 channels to retain more water. Therefore, these patients cannot remove enough water and results in worsening serum dilution and hypoosmolarity [98]. All this mechanism gives place to dilutional hyponatremia, which is the commonest form of hyponatremia in patients with cirrhosis.

In patients hospitalized with cirrhosis and ascites, the prevalence of hyponatremia, defined by sodium <135 mEq/L, is about 22%, which rises to 49% if the cut-off point is 130 mEq/L. The presence of hyponatremia implies a poor prognosis. It has been demonstrated that hyponatremia is an independent predictive factor to have an increased morbidity and mortality and has been added to the MELD score (Sodium-MELD) for liver donor allocation in the United States [99]. When there is a decrease of 1 unit of sodium below 135 mEq/L, the mortality risk increases by over 10% in patients who are in the list for liver transplant [100]. In addition, it has been demonstrated that hyponatremia is a common event in patients with cirrhosis that may lead to hepatic encephalopathy, with implies a significant decline in quality of life and increased neurological complications throughout liver transplantation. Several transplant centers require correction of hyponatremia prior to liver transplantation, but there is no standard algorithm.

There are several types of hyponatremia. On the one hand, hypervolemic or dilutional hyponatremia as explained previously, and on the other hand, hypovolemic hyponatremia, which is usually secondary to excessive fluid losses from the kidney (overdiuresis secondary to diuretic treatment) or from gastrointestinal tract due to diarrhea. If there is an evidence of dehydration or prerenal azotemia, the treatment in these patients consists in solving the cause with fluid volume expansion replacement. Otherwise, if there is a hypervolemic hyponatremia in the setting of volume overload, it is much more difficult to correct the hyponatremia and for patients to tolerate properly the correction. The therapy consists mainly in water restriction and the increase of free water renal excretion. Daily dietary fluid restriction is recommended to 1.5 L, particularly when the serum sodium is below 130 mEq/L. The main drawback of this strategy is the poor patient's compliance and low response. Another point in the treatment is the diuretic adjustment or withdrawal if it is required.

A study of 997 patients with cirrhosis and ascites demonstrated that serum sodium is less than or equal to 120 mmol/L in only 1.2% of patients and less than or equal to 125 mmol/L in only 5.7% [101]. Attempts to rapidly correct hyponatremia in this setting with hypertonic saline can lead to more complications than the hyponatremia itself [2]. Fluid restriction (i.e., 1–1.5 L of water per day) is seldom effective in improving hyponatremia, but prevents a further decrease in sodium levels [2, 3].

There are other strategies under investigation such as increasing the effective arterial blood volume with intravenous albumin with or without vasoconstrictors as, for example, midodrine. These studies are nonrandomized, and there is a need of further studies before their incorporation into clinical practice [102]. Another interesting treatment option for dilutional hyponatremia is the use of vaptans. They induce the release of solute-free water into urine and improve hyponatremia in patients with cirrhosis [103, 104]. Vaptans result useful and effective in improving sodium levels in 45–82% of patients with dilutional hyponatremia. However, the effect is short and goes back to baseline hyponatremia after the withdrawal of the drug, and they do not improve survival. The side effects of this drug are dehydration, thirst, AKI, and overcorrection of sodium levels. Experts in the issue recommend the use of vaptans for a short period of time in patients with hyponatremia below 125 mEq/L who are hospitalized waiting for a liver transplant. Although they have been approved by the Food and Drug Administration and the European Medication Agency for the management of hypervolemic hyponatremia, their widespread use in cirrhosis warrants further long-term studies [2].

7. Hepatorenal syndrome (HRS)

Finally, the last important complication related with ascites is the development of a harmful event such as HRS. HRS is a late manifestation of extreme circulatory dysfunction with a marked vasoconstriction of the kidney arteries trying to compensate splanchnic vasodilatation secondary to portal hypertension. HRS usually appears in patients with cirrhosis and advance stage of liver dysfunction, and it is always accompanied by ascites and usually hyponatremia [105].

HRS may appear with or without precipitating factors, and there are several predictive factors for the development of HRS. The development of bacterial infections, particularly SBP, is the most important risk factor for HRS (30%) [106]. Other important causes include infections, hypovolemia, paracentesis, and bleeding and nephrotoxic medication. HRS is a potentially reversible functional renal impairment in patients with cirrhosis. It may be rapidly progressive (type I HRS) or may develop gradually (type II HRS), which is usually associated with refractory ascites [106]. HRS is diagnosed with clinical and analytical data and its definition has been updated recently. Since the first definition of HRS type 1 in 1994, there have been slight changes, the last one being in 2015 in the revised consensus recommendations of the International Club of Ascites (ICA) [93]. This last change has been made adopting the concept of AKI originally developed in general critically ill patients and has removed the high cut-off value of serum creatinine (2.5 mg/dL or 220 μmol/L) to start pharmacological treatment with vasoconstrictors. HRS type 1 is defined when AKI stage 2 or more is fulfilled with the rest of HRS criteria (see **Table 3**) [80]. In this way, vasoconstrictors and albumin can be administrated earlier and thus potentially achieving a better efficacy. Although this new definition could have benefits in the efficacy, there is still a lack of biomarkers to differentiate between HRS and parenchymal kidney disease such as acute tubular necrosis. The adequate differentiation could select patients with a real functional damage to start the correct treatment as soon as possible. Recently, there are several urine biomarkers under study, trying to help in this hard work.

The prognosis of HRS remains poor, with an average median survival time of nearly 3 months. High MELD scores and type 1 HRS are associated with very poor prognosis. Median survival of patients with untreated type 1 HRS is approximately 1 month [107]. Current guidelines from the European Association for the Study of the Liver emphasize the early detection and treatment of HRS and give priority to liver transplantation [2].

• Diagnosis of cirrhosis with the presence of ascites
• Acute kidney injury stage 2 or more following the International Ascites Club—Acute kidney criteria
• No response to the withdrawal of diuretics and albumin expansion for 48 h
• Absence of shock
• Absence of nephrotoxic drugs in the recent days
• Absence of structural kidney damage evaluated with hematuria >50 hematites/camp, proteinuria >500 mg/day, and normal kidney ultrasonography

Table 3. Hepatorenal syndrome criteria [93].

7.1. Clinical and pharmacological treatment

7.1.1. Terlipressin and norepinephrine

Diuretics should be removed and albumin expansion (1 g/kg) for 48 hours must be administrated if there is no contraindication. If there is no response and the rest of HRS criteria are fulfilled, these patients should be admitted to an intensive care unit. Fluid balance, arterial pressure, vital signs, and central venous pressure are ideally required to prevent volume overload. Current standard treatment involves the use of vasoconstrictors therapy: Terlipressin (1 mg/4–6 hours intravenous bolus) with albumin (20–40 g/day) should be considered as the first-line treatment, and if not available, norepinephrine is a valid alternative. A recent study demonstrated that the administration of terlipressin in continuous infusion instead of boluses had the same rate of response and less side effects [108]. Seventy-eight patients were randomly assigned to receive either continuous intravenous infusion (2 mg/day) or intravenous boluses (0.5 mg/4 h), and if there was no response, the dose was progressively increased to a final dose of 12 mg/day in both groups. The rate of side effects was lower in the infusion than in the boluses (35.29 vs. 62.16%, respectively, $p < 0.025$). The rate of HRS reversal (total and partial) was not significantly different in both groups (76.47 vs. 64.85%). This standard treatment with vasoconstrictor and albumin is effective in 40–50% approximately, although in the last study explained previously it was about 70%. The recurrence of HRS after stopping the vasoconstrictor is about 40%. There are a few studies assessing independent predictive factors of response to terlipressin, and these studies showed a relationship between the improvement in systemic hemodynamics and the effectiveness of treatment. In a study performed in Barcelona, patients with an increase in mean arterial pressure (MAP) of at least 5 mm Hg at day 3 after the beginning of terlipressin, had a higher rate of response. In addition to the improvement in hemodynamics, the degree of liver dysfunction, evaluated with bilirubin greater than 10 mg/dL, was related to a poor response to terlipressin [109]. Another study performed in United States showed that baseline serum creatinine before the beginning of terlipressin predicted the resolution of HRS, and with this information they suggested that an earlier start of treatment would be more effective [110].

A recent RCT compared norepinephrine with terlipressin and demonstrated that reversal of HRS was similar to terlipressin (43 vs. 39%, respectively). Furthermore, there was no statistical difference in survival in both arms: 39% in norepinephrine group and 48% in terlipressin group ($p = 0.461$) [111]. In addition, a recent meta-analysis of 152 patients suggested that norepinephrine is also an effective option for the treatment of HRS as good as terlipressin, when is used in combination with albumin [112].

7.1.2. Midodrine and octreotide

Other therapeutic option is the combination of midodrine and octreotide plus albumin. This therapeutic option has been used widely in countries where terlipressin is not available. A RCT has demonstrated a worse response rate in patients treated with midodrine and octreotide compared to the arm treated with terlipressin (5 vs. 56%, respectively. $p < 0.001$). Ninety-day survival was also lower in the midodrine and octreotide group (29 vs. 56%, $p < 0.06$) [113].

To summarize all these data, although norepinephrine requires an intensive care unit for its use, it is an effective alternative to terlipressin for the treatment of HRS. On the other side, the combination of midodrine and octreotide is not an effective treatment.

7.1.3. Transjugular intrahepatic portosystemic shunt (TIPS)

Transjugular intrahepatic portosystemic shunt (TIPS) may be considered as a second-line therapy, although there is weak evidence to support its use in this complication [2]. TIPS is usually contraindicated in patients with HRS because the syndrome appears in the setting of advanced liver dysfunction. Few small trials have shown renal function improvement and a decrease in renin, aldosterone, and norepinephrine levels after the TIPS insertion [114, 115]. However, data is not strong enough to recommend its use in clinical practice.

7.1.4. Renal replacement therapy

Renal replacement therapy is recommended in guidelines when everything fails, but implies an even worse prognosis [2, 3, 107]. In clinical practice, it is used in patients awaiting liver transplantation, whose renal function did not respond to vasoconstrictor treatment.

7.1.5. Molecular adsorbent recirculating system (MARS)

Liver support with molecular adsorbent recirculating system (MARS) has been used in studies with small sample size in patients who did not respond to standard treatment and it was not effective in changing systemic hemodynamics and kidney function [116]. Only one trial showed a decrease in serum creatinine and bilirubin levels in the arm treated with MARS in comparison to hemodialysis arm [117].

All these invasive treatments are controversially recommended to use in patients without the possibility of liver transplantation and should only be assessed in patients awaiting liver transplant.

7.2. Prevention of HRS

As previously, HRS can be avoided in several situations. The first situation that HRS could be avoided is in large volume paracentesis (LVP). We must give 6-8g of albumin/liter of ascites removed. This action will prevent worsening of circulatory dysfunction, and second, renal impairment, in addition, it also improves survival [2].

The second situation to prevent HRS is in the scenario of SBP. It could be prevented with primary prophylaxis with norfloxacin. Fernandez et al. showed that norfloxacin administration reduced the development of HRS (28 vs. 41%, $p < 0.001$) and 3-month mortality (94 vs. 62%, $p = 0.003$). In addition, norfloxacin administration reduced the 1-year probability of developing a SBP (7 vs. 61%, $p < 0.001$) compared to placebo [83]. Therefore, primary prophylaxis with norfloxacin has an outstanding impact in the clinical course of patients with cirrhosis, reduces the incidence of SBP, delays de development of HRS, and improves survival. This effect is probably secondary to the reduction of bacterial products in the gut, and hence reducing bacterial translocation.

As explained previously, SBP can trigger a kidney failure, which implies a fatal prognosis. In this situation, the utilization of intravenous albumin infusion may improve the effect on circulatory dysfunction in this setting. The study in the Hospital Clinic of Barcelona showed a better 3-month-survival (41 vs. 22%, $p = 0.03$) and lower incidence of kidney failure in patients treated with albumin. (10 vs. 33%, $p = 0.002$). There are ongoing studies, and others done previously recommending the use of albumin expansion in patients with other infections different from SBP, but there is no enough evidence to recommend it in the current guidelines [118].

Author details

Patricia Huelin, Jose Ignacio Fortea, Javier Crespo and Emilio Fábrega*

*Address all correspondence to: digfge@humv.es

Gastroenterology and Hepatology Department, Marqués de Valdecilla University Hospital, Infection, Immunity and Digestive Pathology Group, Research Institute Marqués de Valdecilla (IDIVAL), Grupo Clínico Vinculado al Centro de Investigación Biomédica en Enfermedades Hepáticas y Digestivas (CIBEREHD), Santander, Spain

References

[1] Gines P, Quintero E, Arroyo V, Teres J, Bruguera M, Rimola A, et al. Compensated cirrhosis: Natural history and prognostic factors. Hepatology. 1987;**7**(1):122-128. DOI: 10.1002/hep.1840070124

[2] European Association for the Study of the Liver. EASL clinical practice guidelines on the management of ascites, spontaneous bacterial peritonitis, and hepatorenal syndrome in cirrhosis. Journal of Hepatology. 2010;**53**(3):397-417. DOI: 10.1016/j.jhep.2010.05.004

[3] Runyon BA. Introduction to the revised American Association for the Study of Liver Diseases Practice Guideline management of adult patients with ascites due to cirrhosis 2012. Hepatology. 2013;**57**(4):1651-1653. DOI: 10.1002/hep.26359

[4] Ripoll C, Groszmann R, Garcia-Tsao G, Grace N, Burroughs A, Planas R, et al. Hepatic venous pressure gradient predicts clinical decompensation in patients with compensated cirrhosis. Gastroenterology. 2007;**133**(2):481-488. DOI: 10.1053/j.gastro.2007.05.024

[5] Schrier RW, Arroyo V, Bernardi M, Epstein M, Henriksen JH, Rodes J. Peripheral arterial vasodilation hypothesis: A proposal for the initiation of renal sodium and water retention in cirrhosis. Hepatology. 1988;**8**(5):1151-1157. DOI: 10.1002/hep.1840080532

[6] Fabrega E, Berja A, Garcia-Unzueta MT, Guerra-Ruiz A, Cobo M, Lopez M, et al. Influence of aquaporin-1 gene polymorphism on water retention in liver cirrhosis. Scandinavian Journal of Gastroenterology. 2011;**46**(10):1267-1274. DOI: 10.3109/00365521.2011.603161

[7] Tandon P, Garcia-Tsao G. Bacterial infections, sepsis, and multiorgan failure in cirrhosis. Seminars in Liver Disease. 2008;**28**(1):26-42. DOI: 10.1055/s-2008-1040319

[8] Arroyo V, Gines P, Planas R, Panes J, Rodes J. Management of patients with cirrhosis and ascites. Seminars in Liver Disease. 1986;**6**(4):353-369. DOI: 10.1055/s-2008-1040617

[9] Cardenas A, Arroyo V. Management of ascites and hepatic hydrothorax. Best Practice & Research Clinical Gastroenterology. 2007;**21**(1):55-75. DOI: 10.1016/j.bpg.2006.07.012

[10] Cattau EL Jr, Benjamin SB, Knuff TE, Castell DO. The accuracy of the physical examination in the diagnosis of suspected ascites. JAMA. 1982;**247**(8):1164-1166. DOI: 10.1001/jama.1982.03320330060027

[11] Pose E, Cardenas A. Translating our current understanding of ascites management into new therapies for patients with cirrhosis and fluid retention. Digestive Diseases. 2017;**35**(4):402-410. DOI: 10.1159/000456595

[12] Northup PG, Caldwell SH. Coagulation in liver disease: A guide for the clinician. Clinical Gastroenterology and Hepatology. 2013;**11**(9):1064-1074. DOI: 10.1016/j.cgh.2013.02.026

[13] Grabau CM, Crago SF, Hoff LK, Simon JA, Melton CA, Ott BJ, et al. Performance standards for therapeutic abdominal paracentesis. Hepatology. 2004;**40**(2):484-488. DOI: 10.1002/hep.20317

[14] Runyon BA, Montano AA, Akriviadis EA, Antillon MR, Irving MA, McHutchison JG. The serum-ascites albumin gradient is superior to the exudate-transudate concept in the differential diagnosis of ascites. Annals of Internal Medicine. 1992;**117**(3):215-220. DOI: 10.7326/0003-4819-117-3-215

[15] Runyon BA, Hoefs JC, Morgan TR. Ascitic fluid analysis in malignancy-related ascites. Hepatology. 1988;**8**(5):1104-1109. DOI: 10.1002/hep.1840080521

[16] Wu SS, Lin OS, Chen YY, Hwang KL, Soon MS, Keeffe EB. Ascitic fluid carcinoembryonic antigen and alkaline phosphatase levels for the differentiation of primary from secondary bacterial peritonitis with intestinal perforation. Journal of Hepatology. 2001;**34**(2):215-221. DOI: 10.1016/S0168-8278(00)00039-8

[17] Moore KP, Wong F, Gines P, Bernardi M, Ochs A, Salerno F, et al. The management of ascites in cirrhosis: Report on the consensus conference of the International Ascites Club. Hepatology. 2003;**38**(1):258-266. DOI: 10.1053/jhep.2003.50315

[18] Bernardi M, Laffi G, Salvagnini M, Azzena G, Bonato S, Marra F, et al. Efficacy and safety of the stepped care medical treatment of ascites in liver cirrhosis: A randomized controlled clinical trial comparing two diets with different sodium content. Liver. 1993;**13**(3):156-162. DOI: 10.1111/j.1600-0676.1993.tb00624.x

[19] Salerno F, Guevara M, Bernardi M, Moreau R, Wong F, Angeli P, et al. Refractory ascites: Pathogenesis, definition and therapy of a severe complication in patients with cirrhosis. Liver International. 2010;**30**(7):937-947. DOI: 10.1111/j.1478-3231.2010.02272.x

[20] El-Bokl MA, Senousy BE, El-Karmouty KZ, Mohammed Iel K, Mohammed SM, Shabana SS, et al. Spot urinary sodium for assessing dietary sodium restriction in cirrhotic ascites. World Journal of Gastroenterology. 2009;**15**(29):3631-3635. DOI: 10.3748/wjg.15.3631

[21] Elia C, Graupera I, Barreto R, Sola E, Moreira R, Huelin P, et al. Severe acute kidney injury associated with non-steroidal anti-inflammatory drugs in cirrhosis: A case-control study. Journal of Hepatology. 2015;**63**(3):593-600. DOI: 10.1016/j.jhep.2015.04.004

[22] Garcia-Tsao G, Abraldes JG, Berzigotti A, Bosch J. Portal hypertensive bleeding in cirrhosis: Risk stratification, diagnosis, and management: 2016 practice guidance by the American Association for the study of liver diseases. Hepatology. 2017;**65**(1):310-335. DOI: 10.1002/hep.28906

[23] Romanelli RG, La Villa G, Barletta G, Vizzutti F, Lanini F, Arena U, et al. Long-term albumin infusion improves survival in patients with cirrhosis and ascites: An unblinded randomized trial. World Journal of Gastroenterology. 2006;**12**(9):1403-1407. DOI: 10.3748/wjg.v12.i9.1403.

[24] EASL Clinical Practice Guidelines: Liver transplantation. Journal of Hepatology. 2016;**64**(2):433-485. DOI: 10.1016/j.jhep.2015.10.006

[25] Lenz K, Buder R, Kapun L, Voglmayr M. Treatment and management of ascites and hepatorenal syndrome: An update. Therapeutic Advances in Gastroenterology. 2015;**8**(2):83-100. DOI: 10.1177/1756283x14564673

[26] Kao HW, Rakov NE, Savage E, Reynolds TB. The effect of large volume paracentesis on plasma volume – a cause of hypovolemia? Hepatology. 1985;**5**(3):403-407. DOI: 10.1002/hep.1840050310

[27] Annamalai A, Wisdom L, Herada M, Nourredin M, Ayoub W, Sundaram V, et al. Management of refractory ascites in cirrhosis: Are we out of date? World Journal of Hepatology. 2016;**8**(28):1182-1193. DOI: 10.4254/wjh.v8.i28.1182

[28] Bernardi M, Caraceni P, Navickis RJ, Wilkes MM. Albumin infusion in patients undergoing large-volume paracentesis: A meta-analysis of randomized trials. Hepatology. 2012;**55**(4):1172-1181. DOI: 10.1002/hep.24786

[29] Alessandria C, Elia C, Mezzabotta L, Risso A, Andrealli A, Spandre M, et al. Prevention of paracentesis-induced circulatory dysfunction in cirrhosis: Standard vs. half albumin doses. A prospective, randomized, unblinded pilot study. Digestive and Liver Disease. 2011;**43**(11):881-886. DOI: 10.1016/j.dld.2011.06.001

[30] Boyer TD, Haskal ZJ. The role of Transjugular Intrahepatic Portosystemic Shunt (TIPS) in the Management of Portal Hypertension: Update 2009. Hepatology. 2010;**51**(1):306. DOI: 10.1002/hep.23383

[31] Gines P, Uriz J, Calahorra B, Garcia-Tsao G, Kamath PS, Del Arbol LR, et al. Transjugular intrahepatic portosystemic shunting versus paracentesis plus albumin for refractory ascites in cirrhosis. Gastroenterology. 2002;**123**(6):1839-1847. DOI: 10.1053/gast.2002.37073

[32] Narahara Y, Kanazawa H, Fukuda T, Matsushita Y, Harimoto H, Kidokoro H, et al. Transjugular intrahepatic portosystemic shunt versus paracentesis plus albumin in patients with refractory ascites who have good hepatic and renal function: A prospective randomized trial. Journal of Gastroenterology. 2011;**46**(1):78-85. DOI: 10.1007/s00535-010-0282-9

[33] Salerno F, Merli M, Riggio O, Cazzaniga M, Valeriano V, Pozzi M, et al. Randomized controlled study of TIPS versus paracentesis plus albumin in cirrhosis with severe ascites. Hepatology. 2004;**40**(3):629-635. DOI: 10.1002/hep.20364

[34] Bureau C, Thabut D, Oberti F, Dharancy S, Carbonell N, Bouvier A, et al. Transjugular intrahepatic portosystemic shunts with covered stents increase transplant-free survival of patients with cirrhosis and recurrent ascites. Gastroenterology. 2017;**152**(1):157-163. DOI: 10.1053/j.gastro.2016.09.016

[35] Lebrec D, Giuily N, Hadengue A, Vilgrain V, Moreau R, Poynard T, et al. Transjugular intrahepatic portosystemic shunts: Comparison with paracentesis in patients with cirrhosis and refractory ascites: A randomized trial. French Group of Clinicians and a Group of Biologists. Journal of Hepatology. 1996;**25**(2):135-144. DOI: 10.1016/S0168-8278(96)80065-1

[36] Rossle M, Ochs A, Gulberg V, Siegerstetter V, Holl J, Deibert P, et al. A comparison of paracentesis and transjugular intrahepatic portosystemic shunting in patients with ascites. The New England Journal of Medicine. 2000;**342**(23):1701-1707. DOI: 10.1056/nejm200006083422303

[37] Sanyal AJ, Genning C, Reddy KR, Wong F, Kowdley KV, Benner K, et al. The North American study for the treatment of refractory ascites. Gastroenterology. 2003;**124**(3):634-641. DOI: 10.1053/gast.2003.50088

[38] Albillos A, Banares R, Gonzalez M, Catalina MV, Molinero LM. A meta-analysis of transjugular intrahepatic portosystemic shunt versus paracentesis for refractory ascites. Journal of Hepatology. 2005;**43**(6):990-996. DOI: 10.1016/j.jhep.2005.06.005

[39] D'Amico G, Luca A, Morabito A, Miraglia R, D'Amico M. Uncovered transjugular intrahepatic portosystemic shunt for refractory ascites: A meta-analysis. Gastroenterology. 2005;**129**(4):1282-1293. DOI: 10.1053/j.gastro.2005.07.031

[40] Deltenre P, Mathurin P, Dharancy S, Moreau R, Bulois P, Henrion J, et al. Transjugular intrahepatic portosystemic shunt in refractory ascites: A meta-analysis. Liver International. 2005;**25**(2):349-356. DOI: 10.1111/j.1478-3231.2005.01095.x

[41] Saab S, Nieto JM, Lewis SK, Runyon BA. TIPS versus paracentesis for cirrhotic patients with refractory ascites. The Cochrane Database of Systematic Reviews. 2006(4):Cd004889. DOI: 10.1002/14651858.CD004889.pub2

[42] Salerno F, Camma C, Enea M, Rossle M, Wong F. Transjugular intrahepatic portosystemic shunt for refractory ascites: A meta-analysis of individual patient data. Gastroenterology. 2007;**133**(3):825-834. DOI: 10.1053/j.gastro.2007.06.020

[43] Bai M, Qi XS, Yang ZP, Yang M, Fan DM, Han GH. TIPS improves liver transplantation-free survival in cirrhotic patients with refractory ascites: An updated meta-analysis. World Journal of Gastroenterology. 2014;**20**(10):2704-2714. DOI: 10.3748/wjg.v20.i10.2704

[44] Rossle M. TIPS: 25 years later. Journal of Hepatology. 2013;**59**(5):1081-1093. DOI: 10.1016/j.jhep.2013.06.014

[45] Fagiuoli S, Bruno R, Debernardi Venon W, Schepis F, Vizzutti F, Toniutto P, et al. Consensus conference on TIPS management: Techniques, indications, contraindications. Digestive and Liver Disease. 2017;**49**(2):121-137. DOI: 10.1016/j.dld.2016.10.011

[46] Smith M, Durham J. Evolving Indications for Tips. Techniques in Vascular and Interventional Radiology. 2016;**19**(1):36-41. DOI: 10.1053/j.tvir.2016.01.004

[47] Stirnimann G, Banz V, Storni F, De Gottardi A. Automated low-flow ascites pump for the treatment of cirrhotic patients with refractory ascites. Therapeutic Advances in Gastroenterology. 2017;**10**(2):283-292. DOI: 10.1177/1756283x16684688

[48] Bureau C, Adebayo D, de Rieu MC, Elkrief L, Valla D, Peck-Radosavljevic M, et al. Alfapump system vs. large volume paracentesis for refractory ascites: A multicenter randomized controlled study. Journal of Hepatology. 2017. In press

[49] Bellot P, Welker MW, Soriano G, von Schaewen M, Appenrodt B, Wiest R, et al. Automated low flow pump system for the treatment of refractory ascites: A multi-center safety and efficacy study. Journal of Hepatology. 2013;**58**(5):922-927. DOI: 10.1016/j.jhep.2012.12.020

[50] Sola E, Sanchez-Cabus S, Rodriguez E, Elia C, Cela R, Moreira R, et al. Effects of alfapump system on kidney and circulatory function in patients with cirrhosis and refractory ascites. Liver Transplantation. 2017;**23**(5):583-593. DOI: 10.1002/lt.24763

[51] Wong F, Gines P, Watson H, Horsmans Y, Angeli P, Gow P, et al. Effects of a selective vasopressin V2 receptor antagonist, satavaptan, on ascites recurrence after paracentesis in patients with cirrhosis. Journal of Hepatology. 2010;**53**(2):283-290. DOI: 10.1016/j.jhep.2010.02.036

[52] Wong F, Watson H, Gerbes A, Vilstrup H, Badalamenti S, Bernardi M, et al. Satavaptan for the management of ascites in cirrhosis: Efficacy and safety across the spectrum of ascites severity. Gut. 2012;**61**(1):108-116. DOI: 10.1136/gutjnl-2011-300157

[53] Sakaida I, Yamashita S, Kobayashi T, Komatsu M, Sakai T, Komorizono Y, et al. Efficacy and safety of a 14-day administration of tolvaptan in the treatment of patients with ascites in hepatic oedema. Journal of International Medical Research. 2013;**41**(3):835-847. DOI: 10.1177/0300060513480089

[54] Zhang X, Wang SZ, Zheng JF, Zhao WM, Li P, Fan CL, et al. Clinical efficacy of tolvaptan for treatment of refractory ascites in liver cirrhosis patients. World Journal of Gastroenterology. 2014;**20**(32):11400-11405. DOI: 10.3748/wjg.v20.i32.11400

[55] Akiyama S, Ikeda K, Sezaki H, Fukushima T, Sorin Y, Kawamura Y, et al. Therapeutic effects of short- and intermediate-term tolvaptan administration for refractory ascites in patients with advanced liver cirrhosis. Hepatology Research. 2015;**45**(11):1062-1070. DOI: 10.1111/hepr.12455

[56] Ohki T, Sato K, Yamada T, Yamagami M, Ito D, Kawanishi K, et al. Efficacy of tolvaptan in patients with refractory ascites in a clinical setting. World Journal of Hepatology. 2015;**7**(12):1685-1693. DOI: 10.4254/wjh.v7.i12.1685

[57] Chishina H, Hagiwara S, Nishida N, Ueshima K, Sakurai T, Ida H, et al. Clinical factors predicting the effect of tolvaptan for refractory ascites in patients with decompensated liver cirrhosis. Digestive Diseases. 2016;**34**(6):659-664. DOI: 10.1159/000448828

[58] Sakaida I, Kawazoe S, Kajimura K, Saito T, Okuse C, Takaguchi K, et al. Tolvaptan for improvement of hepatic edema: A phase 3, multicenter, randomized, double-blind, placebo-controlled trial. Hepatology Research. 2014;**44**(1):73-82. DOI: 10.1111/hepr.12098

[59] Okita K, Kawazoe S, Hasebe C, Kajimura K, Kaneko A, Okada M, et al. Dose-finding trial of tolvaptan in liver cirrhosis patients with hepatic edema: A randomized, double-blind, placebo-controlled trial. Hepatology Research. 2014;**44**(1):83-91. DOI: 10.1111/hepr.12099

[60] Cardenas A, Gines P, Marotta P, Czerwiec F, Oyuang J, Guevara M, et al. Tolvaptan, an oral vasopressin antagonist, in the treatment of hyponatremia in cirrhosis. Journal of Hepatology. 2012;**56**(3):571-578. DOI: 10.1016/j.jhep.2011.08.020

[61] Torres VE, Chapman AB, Devuyst O, Gansevoort RT, Grantham JJ, Higashihara E, et al. Tolvaptan in patients with autosomal dominant polycystic kidney disease. The New England Journal of Medicine. 2012;**367**(25):2407-2418. DOI: 10.1056/NEJMoa1205511

[62] Angeli P, Volpin R, Piovan D, Bortoluzzi A, Craighero R, Bottaro S, et al. Acute effects of the oral administration of midodrine, an alpha-adrenergic agonist, on renal hemodynamics and renal function in cirrhotic patients with ascites. Hepatology. 1998;**28**(4):937-943. DOI: 10.1002/hep.510280407

[63] Kalambokis G, Fotopoulos A, Economou M, Pappas K, Tsianos EV. Effects of a 7-day treatment with midodrine in non-azotemic cirrhotic patients with and without ascites. Journal of Hepatology. 2007;**46**(2):213-221. DOI: 10.1016/j.jhep.2006.09.012

[64] Kalambokis G, Economou M, Fotopoulos A, Al Bokharhii J, Pappas C, Katsaraki A, et al. The effects of chronic treatment with octreotide versus octreotide plus midodrine on systemic hemodynamics and renal hemodynamics and function in nonazotemic cirrhotic patients with ascites. The American Journal of Gastroenterology. 2005;**100**(4):879-885. DOI: 10.1111/j.1572-0241.2005.40899.x

[65] Singh V, Dhungana SP, Singh B, Vijayverghia R, Nain CK, Sharma N, et al. Midodrine in patients with cirrhosis and refractory or recurrent ascites: A randomized pilot study. Journal of Hepatology. 2012;**56**(2):348-354. DOI: 10.1016/j.jhep.2011.04.027

[66] Rai N, Singh B, Singh A, Vijayvergiya R, Sharma N, Bhalla A, et al. Midodrine and tolvaptan in patients with cirrhosis and refractory or recurrent ascites: A randomised pilot study. Liver International. 2017;**37**(3):406-414. DOI: 10.1111/liv.13250

[67] Lenaerts A, Van Cauter J, Moukaiber H, Meunier JC, Ligny G. Treatment of refractory ascites with clonidine and spironolactone. Gastroentérologie Clinique et Biologique. 1997;**21**(6-7):524-525. DOI: 10.1016/S1879-8551(16)49558-8

[68] Lenaerts A, Codden T, Van Cauter J, Meunier JC, Henry JP, Ligny G. Interest of the association clonidine-spironolactone in cirrhotic patients with ascites and activation of sympathetic nervous system. Acta Gastro-Enterologica Belgica. 2002;**65**(1):1-5

[69] Lenaerts A, Codden T, Meunier JC, Henry JP, Ligny G. Effects of clonidine on diuretic response in ascitic patients with cirrhosis and activation of sympathetic nervous system. Hepatology. 2006;**44**(4):844-849. DOI: 10.1002/hep.21355

[70] Yang YY, Lin HC, Lee WP, Chu CJ, Lin MW, Lee FY, et al. Association of the G-protein and alpha2-adrenergic receptor gene and plasma norepinephrine level with clonidine improvement of the effects of diuretics in patients with cirrhosis with refractory ascites: A randomised clinical trial. Gut. 2010;**59**(11):1545-1553. DOI: 10.1136/gut.2010.210732

[71] Singh V, Singh A, Singh B, Vijayvergiya R, Sharma N, Ghai A, et al. Midodrine and clonidine in patients with cirrhosis and refractory or recurrent ascites: A randomized pilot study. The American Journal of Gastroenterology. 2013;**108**(4):560-567. DOI: 10.1038/ajg.2013.9

[72] Krag A, Moller S, Henriksen JH, Holstein-Rathlou NH, Larsen FS, Bendtsen F. Terlipressin improves renal function in patients with cirrhosis and ascites without hepatorenal syndrome. Hepatology. 2007;**46**(6):1863-1871. DOI: 10.1002/hep.21901

[73] Fimiani B, Guardia DD, Puoti C, D'Adamo G, Cioffi O, Pagano A, et al. The use of terlipressin in cirrhotic patients with refractory ascites and normal renal function: A multicentric study. European Journal of Internal Medicine. 2011;**22**(6):587-590. DOI: 10.1016/j.ejim.2011.06.013

[74] Conn HO. Spontaneous peritonitis and bacteremia in laennec's cirrhosis caused by enteric organisms. A relatively common but rarely recognized syndrome. Annals of Internal Medicine. 1964;**60**:568-580. DOI: 10.7326/0003-4819-60-4-568

[75] Berg RD. Bacterial translocation from the gastrointestinal tract. Advances in Experimental Medicine and Biology. 1999;**473**:11-30. DOI: 10.1016/S0966-842X(00)88906-4

[76] Moreau R, Jalan R, Gines P, Pavesi M, Angeli P, Cordoba J, et al. Acute-on-chronic liver failure is a distinct syndrome that develops in patients with acute decompensation of cirrhosis. Gastroenterology. 2013;**144**(7):1426-1437. e1-9. DOI: 10.1053/j.gastro.2013.02.042

[77] Follo A, Llovet JM, Navasa M, Planas R, Forns X, Francitorra A, et al. Renal impairment after spontaneous bacterial peritonitis in cirrhosis: Incidence, clinical course, predictive factors and prognosis. Hepatology. 1994;**20**(6):1495-1501. DOI: 10.1002/hep.1840200619

[78] Fernandez J, Acevedo J, Castro M, Garcia O, de Lope CR, Roca D, et al. Prevalence and risk factors of infections by multiresistant bacteria in cirrhosis: A prospective study. Hepatology. 2012;**55**(5):1551-1561. DOI: 10.1002/hep.25532

[79] Moore KP, Aithal GP. Guidelines on the management of ascites in cirrhosis. Gut. 2006;**55**(Suppl 6):vi1-vi12. DOI: 10.1136/gut.2006.099580

[80] Sort P, Navasa M, Arroyo V, Aldeguer X, Planas R, Ruiz-del-Arbol L, et al. Effect of intravenous albumin on renal impairment and mortality in patients with cirrhosis and spontaneous bacterial peritonitis. The New England Journal of Medicine. 1999;**341**(6):403-409. DOI: 10.1056/nejm199908053410603

[81] Arroyo V, Fernandez J. Management of hepatorenal syndrome in patients with cirrhosis. Nature Reviews Nephrology. 2011;**7**(9):517-526. DOI: 10.1038/nrneph.2011.96

[82] Guarner C, Sola R, Soriano G, Andreu M, Novella MT, Vila MC, et al. Risk of a first community-acquired spontaneous bacterial peritonitis in cirrhotic with low ascitic fluid protein levels. Gastroenterology. 1999;**117**(2):414-419. DOI: 10.1053/gast.1999.0029900414

[83] Fernandez J, Navasa M, Planas R, Montoliu S, Monfort D, Soriano G, et al. Primary prophylaxis of spontaneous bacterial peritonitis delays hepatorenal syndrome and improves survival in cirrhosis. Gastroenterology. 2007;**133**(3):818-824. DOI: 10.1053/j.gastro.2007.06.065

[84] Akriviadis EA, Runyon BA. Utility of an algorithm in differentiating spontaneous from secondary bacterial peritonitis. Gastroenterology. 1990;**98**(1):127-133.

[85] Soriano G, Castellote J, Alvarez C, Girbau A, Gordillo J, Baliellas C, et al. Secondary bacterial peritonitis in cirrhosis: A retrospective study of clinical and analytical characteristics, diagnosis and management. Journal of Hepatology. 2010;**52**(1):39-44. DOI: 10.1016/j.jhep.2009.10.012

[86] Ariza X, Castellote J, Lora-Tamayo J, Girbau A, Salord S, Rota R, et al. Risk factors for resistance to ceftriaxone and its impact on mortality in community, healthcare and nosocomial spontaneous bacterial peritonitis. Journal of Hepatology. 2012;**56**(4):825-832. DOI: 10.1016/j.jhep.2011.11.010

[87] Fernandez J, Navasa M, Gomez J, Colmenero J, Vila J, Arroyo V, et al. Bacterial infections in cirrhosis: Epidemiological changes with invasive procedures and norfloxacin prophylaxis. Hepatology. 2002;**35**(1):140-148. DOI: 10.1053/jhep.2002.30082

[88] Piano S, Romano A, Rosi S, Gatta A, Angeli P. Spontaneous bacterial peritonitis due to carbapenemase-producing *Klebsiella pneumoniae*: The last therapeutic challenge. European Journal of Gastroenterology & Hepatology. 2012;**24**(10):1234-1237. DOI: 10.1097/MEG.0b013e328355d8a2

[89] Piano S, Fasolato S, Salinas F, Romano A, Tonon M, Morando F, et al. The empirical antibiotic treatment of nosocomial spontaneous bacterial peritonitis: Results of a randomized, controlled clinical trial. Hepatology. 2016;**63**(4):1299-1309. DOI: 10.1002/hep.27941

[90] Gines P, Rimola A, Planas R, Vargas V, Marco F, Almela M, et al. Norfloxacin prevents spontaneous bacterial peritonitis recurrence in cirrhosis: Results of a double-blind, placebo-controlled trial. Hepatology. 1990;**12**(4 Pt 1):716-724. DOI: 10.1002/hep.1840120416

[91] Soriano G, Guarner C, Teixido M, Such J, Barrios J, Enriquez J, et al. Selective intestinal decontamination prevents spontaneous bacterial peritonitis. Gastroenterology. 1991;**100**(2):477-481. DOI: 10.5555/uri:pii:001650859190219B

[92] Jalan R, Fernandez J, Wiest R, Schnabl B, Moreau R, Angeli P, et al. Bacterial infections in cirrhosis: A position statement based on the EASL Special Conference 2013. Journal of Hepatology. 2014;**60**(6):1310-1324. DOI: 10.1016/j.jhep.2014.01.024

[93] Angeli P, Gines P, Wong F, Bernardi M, Boyer TD, Gerbes A, et al. Diagnosis and management of acute kidney injury in patients with cirrhosis: Revised consensus recommendations of the International Club of Ascites. Gut. 2015;**64**(4):531-537. DOI: 10.1136/gutjnl-2014-308874

[94] Bass NM, Mullen KD, Sanyal A, Poordad F, Neff G, Leevy CB, et al. Rifaximin treatment in hepatic encephalopathy. The New England Journal of Medicine. 2010;**362**(12):1071-1081. DOI: 10.1056/NEJMoa0907893

[95] Lutz P, Parcina M, Bekeredjian-Ding I, Nischalke HD, Nattermann J, Sauerbruch T, et al. Impact of rifaximin on the frequency and characteristics of spontaneous bacterial peritonitis in patients with liver cirrhosis and ascites. PLoS One. 2014;**9**(4):e93909. DOI: 10.1371/journal.pone.0093909

[96] Elfert A, Abo Ali L, Soliman S, Ibrahim S, Abd-Elsalam S. Randomized-controlled trial of rifaximin versus norfloxacin for secondary prophylaxis of spontaneous bacterial peritonitis. European Journal of Gastroenterology & Hepatology. 2016;**28**(12):1450-1454. DOI: 10.1097/meg.0000000000000724

[97] Gines P, Guevara M. Hyponatremia in cirrhosis: Pathogenesis, clinical significance, and management. Hepatology. 2008;**48**(3):1002-1010. DOI: 10.1002/hep.22418

[98] Lizaola B, Bonder A, Tapper EB, Mendez-Bocanegra A, Cardenas A. The changing role of sodium management in cirrhosis. Current Treatment Options in Gastroenterology. 2016;**14**(2):274-284. DOI: 10.1007/s11938-016-0094-y

[99] Biggins SW, Rodriguez HJ, Bacchetti P, Bass NM, Roberts JP, Terrault NA. Serum sodium predicts mortality in patients listed for liver transplantation. Hepatology. 2005;**41**(1):32-39. DOI: 10.1002/hep.20517

[100] Londono MC, Guevara M, Rimola A, Navasa M, Taura P, Mas A, et al. Hyponatremia impairs early posttransplantation outcome in patients with cirrhosis undergoing liver transplantation. Gastroenterology. 2006;**130**(4):1135-1143. DOI: 10.1053/j.gastro.2006.02.017

[101] Angeli P, Wong F, Watson H, Gines P. Hyponatremia in cirrhosis: Results of a patient population survey. Hepatology. 2006;**44**(6):1535-1542. DOI: 10.1002/hep.21412

[102] McCormick PA, Mistry P, Kaye G, Burroughs AK, McIntyre N. Intravenous albumin infusion is an effective therapy for hyponatremia in cirrhotic patients with ascites. Gut. 1990;**31**(2):204-207. DOI: 10.1136/gut.31.2.204

[103] Schrier RW, Gross P, Gheorghiade M, Berl T, Verbalis JG, Czerwiec FS, et al. Tolvaptan, a selective oral vasopressin V2-receptor antagonist, for hyponatremia. The New England Journal of Medicine. 2006;**355**(20):2099-2112. DOI: 10.1056/NEJMoa065181

[104] Wong F, Blei AT, Blendis LM, Thuluvath PJ. A vasopressin receptor antagonist (VPA-985) improves serum sodium concentration in patients with hyponatremia: A multicenter, randomized, placebo-controlled trial. Hepatology. 2003;**37**(1):182-191. DOI: 10.1053/jhep.2003.50021

[105] Gines P, Schrier RW. Renal failure in cirrhosis. The New England Journal of Medicine. 2009;**361**(13):1279-1290. DOI: 10.1056/NEJMra0809139

[106] Cardenas A, Gines P, Uriz J, Bessa X, Salmeron JM, Mas A, et al. Renal failure after upper gastrointestinal bleeding in cirrhosis: Incidence, clinical course, predictive factors, and short-term prognosis. Hepatology. 2001;**34**(4 Pt 1):671-676. DOI: 10.1053/jhep.2001.27830

[107] Cavallin M, Piano S, Romano A, Fasolato S, Frigo AC, Benetti G, et al. Terlipressin given by continuous intravenous infusion versus intravenous boluses in the treatment of hepatorenal syndrome: A randomized controlled study. Hepatology. 2016;**63**(3):983-992. DOI: 10.1002/hep.28396

[108] Martin-Llahi M, Pepin MN, Guevara M, Diaz F, Torre A, Monescillo A, et al. Terlipressin and albumin vs. albumin in patients with cirrhosis and hepatorenal syndrome: A randomized study. Gastroenterology. 2008;**134**(5):1352-1359. DOI: 10.1053/j.gastro.2008.02.024

[109] Nazar A, Pereira GH, Guevara M, Martin-Llahi M, Pepin MN, Marinelli M, et al. Predictors of response to therapy with terlipressin and albumin in patients with cirrhosis and type 1 hepatorenal syndrome. Hepatology. 2010;**51**(1):219-226. DOI: 10.1002/hep.23283

[110] Boyer TD, Sanyal AJ, Garcia-Tsao G, Blei A, Carl D, Bexon AS, et al. Predictors of response to terlipressin plus albumin in hepatorenal syndrome (HRS) type 1: Relationship of serum creatinine to hemodynamics. Journal of Hepatology. 2011;**55**(2):315-321. DOI: 10.1016/j.jhep.2010.11.020

[111] Singh V, Ghosh S, Singh B, Kumar P, Sharma N, Bhalla A, et al. Noradrenaline vs. terlipressin in the treatment of hepatorenal syndrome: A randomized study. Journal of Hepatology. 2012;**56**(6):1293-1298. DOI: 10.1016/j.jhep.2012.01.012

[112] Nassar Junior AP, Farias AQ, D'Albuquerque LA, Carrilho FJ, Malbouisson LM. Terlipressin versus norepinephrine in the treatment of hepatorenal syndrome: A systematic review and meta-analysis. PLoS One. 2014;**9**(9):e107466. DOI: 10.1371/journal.pone.0107466

[113] Cavallin M, Kamath PS, Merli M, Fasolato S, Toniutto P, Salerno F, et al. Terlipressin plus albumin versus midodrine and octreotide plus albumin in the treatment of hepatorenal syndrome: A randomized trial. Hepatology. 2015;**62**(2):567-574. DOI: 10.1002/hep.27709

[114] Guevara M, Gines P, Bandi JC, Gilabert R, Sort P, Jimenez W, et al. Transjugular intrahepatic portosystemic shunt in hepatorenal syndrome: Effects on renal function and vasoactive systems. Hepatology. 1998;**28**(2):416-422. DOI: 10.1002/hep.510280219

[115] Rossle M, Gerbes AL. TIPS for the treatment of refractory ascites, hepatorenal syndrome and hepatic hydrothorax: A critical update. Gut. 2010;**59**(7):988-1000. DOI: 10.1136/gut.2009.193227

[116] Lavayssiere L, Kallab S, Cardeau-Desangles I, Nogier MB, Cointault O, Barange K, et al. Impact of molecular adsorbent recirculating system on renal recovery in type-1 hepatorenal syndrome patients with chronic liver failure. Journal of Gastroenterology and Hepatology. 2013;**28**(6):1019-1024. DOI: 10.1111/jgh.12159

[117] Wong F, Raina N, Richardson R. Molecular adsorbent recirculating system is ineffective in the management of type 1 hepatorenal syndrome in patients with cirrhosis with ascites who have failed vasoconstrictor treatment. Gut. 2010;**59**(3):381-386. DOI: 10.1136/gut.2008.174615

[118] Guevara M, Terra C, Nazar A, Sola E, Fernandez J, Pavesi M, et al. Albumin for bacterial infections other than spontaneous bacterial peritonitis in cirrhosis. A randomized, controlled study. Journal of Hepatology. 2012;**57**(4):759-765. DOI: 10.1016/j.jhep.2012.06.013

Chapter 6

Pharmacological Therapy of Ascites

Aziza Ajlan, Waleed K. Al-hamoudi and
Hussein Elsiesy

Additional information is available at the end of the chapter

http://dx.doi.org/10.5772/intechopen.70544

Abstract

Ascites refer to accumulation of fluids in the peritoneal cavity. Ascites is caused by multiple causes, among which liver cirrhosis is the commonest. Confirming the etiology is the first and most important step toward proper management. Assuming that ascites is always caused by cirrhosis can lead to unnecessarily sending patients with different etiologies for liver transplantation, particularly patients with non-cirrhotic portal hypertension. Calculating serum albumin ascitic gradient is important in differentiating ascites due to portal hypertension from other etiologies. The first-line therapy for ascites in cirrhosis is low salt diet and diuretics. It is important to avoid nonsteroidal anti-inflammatory drugs (NSAIDs) and nephrotoxic medications in these patients.

Keywords: ascites, treatment, pharmacological therapy, liver cirrhosis

1. Introduction

Even though liver disease remains the main cause of ascites, there are several other causes including renal diseases, infections (tuberculosis), malignancies, and heart disease (**Table 1**).

It is important to diagnose the etiology of ascites in order to properly treat it.

Detailed history, physical examination, laboratory blood test, abdominal ultrasound, and serum albumin ascitic gradient are important in narrowing the differential diagnosis of ascites.

Cirrhosis is the eighth leading cause of death in the United States [1]. Ascites is one of the most common complications of cirrhosis that leads to hospital admissions [2]. It occurs due

High SAAG ascites (>1.1)	Low SAAG ascites (<1.1)
Liver cirrhosis	Tuberculosis
Budd-Chiari syndrome	Malignancy
Sinusoidal obstructive syndrome	Pancreatic
Heart failure (high protein)	Renal
Alcoholic hepatitis	Serositis
Acute liver failure	

Table 1. Causes of ascites.

to portal hypertension and is primarily related to an inability to excrete an adequate amount of sodium into urine, leading to positive sodium balance leading to fluid retention [3]. Many patients are referred for liver transplantation after development of ascites. Evidence suggests that arterial splanchnic vasodilation leads to renal sodium and water retention in patients with cirrhosis. This permits dropping in effective arterial blood capacity with stimulation of arterial as well as cardiopulmonary volume receptors, in addition to homeostatic stimulation of vasoconstrictor and sodium-retaining systems (i.e., the RAAS (renin-angiotensin-aldosterone system) as well as the sympathetic nervous system). Renal sodium preservation causes extension of the extracellular fluid volume and accumulation of ascites and edema [4, 5]. The occurrence of ascites is directly linked to worse prognosis and compromised life quality; therefore, patients should be turned over to liver transplant center for evaluation [6]. Nearly 75% of the patients with ascites in Western Europe or the United States have cirrhosis as the primary cause. The remaining 25% of the ascites is caused by malignancy, heart failure, tuberculosis, pancreatic disease, or other miscellaneous causes [7].

Determining the cause of ascites is very important for appropriate management. The serum-ascites albumin gradient (SAAG) can be helpful for both diagnostic and therapeutic purposes. Patients with a high SAAG (≥1.1 g/dL) have portal hypertension and usually are responsive to diuretic therapy measures [8].

1.1. First-line treatment

One of the most important steps in treating ascites in this setting is to treat the underlying liver disease. In patients with alcoholic liver disease, abstinence from alcohol intake can result in dramatic improvement in the reversible component of alcoholic liver disease. This measure alone can lead to an around 75% 3-year survival. If the patient does not succeed in refraining from alcohol intake, they may die within 3 years [9]. Abstinence from alcohol intake alone may lead to either complete resolution of ascites or at least a better response to medical therapy.

Ascites in decompensated hepatitis B virus infection-related cirrhosis and autoimmune hepatitis can also have a great response to specific drug therapy, although liver disease is unlikely to be revisable by the time ascites is manifested (**Table 2**) [10].

Treatment of ascites due to liver cirrhosis
1. Treatment of the underlying cause: stop alcohol, treat AIH, and HBV
2. Low-salt diet and diuretics
3. Water restriction if sodium <120 mmol
4. Vaptans (not effective)
5. Albumin and colloid replacement
6. Avoid nephrotoxic medications

Table 2. Treatment of ascites due to liver cirrhosis.

2. Diet and diuretics

The first-line treatment of patients with cirrhosis and ascites includes (1) dietary sodium restriction (2000 mg/day [88 mmol/day]) and (2) oral diuretics [11]. Evidence suggests that renal sodium retention in these patients is mainly caused by increased proximal as well as distal tubular sodium reabsorption instead of reduction of filtered sodium load [12, 13]. Although the mechanism by which enhanced proximal tubular reabsorption of sodium occurs has not been fully established, the increased reabsorption of sodium along the distal tubule is mainly due to hyperaldosteronism [14]. Therefore, aldosterone antagonists are considered the treatment of choice and are more effective than loop diuretics. Amiloride (with doses of 10–40 mg/day), a diuretic acting in the collecting duct, is less effective than the active metabolite spironolactone and much more expensive and should be used as an alternative only in those patients who develop side effects with aldosterone antagonists (e.g., tender gynecomastia) [15]. There has been a long argument, whether aldosterone should be administered alone or coupled with loop diuretics. Two studies have assessed both approaches. The first used aldosterone antagonists in a stepwise increase every 7 days (up to 400 mg/day) in combination with furosemide (40–160 mg/day, in 40 mg/day steps) considered only in patients not exhibiting proper response to maximum doses of aldosterone antagonists versus joint treatment of aldosterone antagonists and furosemide from the commencement of treatment (100 in addition to 40 mg/day with the option to build the dose in a stepwise manner every 7 days in view of lack of response up to 400 and 160 mg/day) [16, 17]. The results of the two studies were inconsistent with each other probably due to differences in patient populations, in particular, with regard to the percentage of patients with the first episode of ascites [17]. Initiation of both drugs appears to be the favored approach in attaining quick natriuresis and preserving normokalemia. Single morning dosing enhances adherence. Dosing more than once daily decreases adherence and may lead to nocturia.

The maximum doses are 400 mg/day of spironolactone and 160 mg/day of furosemide [8, 11]. Furosemide can be suspended for a short period of time in patients with hypokalemia, which is very common in the setting of alcoholic hepatitis.

Other diuretics including triamterene, metolazone, and hydrochlorothiazide have also been used to treat ascites [11].

Eplerenone is a newer aldosterone antagonist that has been used in heart failure [18]. There is only one study evaluating the use of eplerenone in ascites with comparable results to aldactone [19]. It could also serve as substitute of spironolactone in patients who develop tender gynecomastia [20].

Other loop diuretics, such as torasemide and bumetanide, are currently not being used as they did not seem to demonstrate superiority to the current agents, let alone their cost.

It's important to mention though, in all patients, diuretic therapy should aim to achieve weight loss of no more than 0.5 kg/day if peripheral edema is absent and 1 kg/day in those with peripheral edema to avoid diuretic-related renal failure and/or hyponatremia which is mainly due to intravascular volume depletion [7]. Other complications of diuretic therapy include hepatic encephalopathy, electrolyte disorders, gynaecomastia, and muscle cramps [13, 21–37]. If cramps are severe, diuretic dose should be decreased or stopped, and albumin infusion [37], baclofen, and L-carnitine may relieve symptoms [23–27, 37].

3. Fluid restriction

Fluid restriction is not necessary in treating most patients with cirrhosis and ascites unless sodium is less than 120. The chronic hyponatremia commonly observed in cirrhotic ascites patients is occasionally fatal if not corrected. One study with 997 cirrhotic patients with ascites showed that the serum sodium is ≤120 mmol/L in 1.2% of the patients and ≤ 125 mmol/L in only 5.7%. Rapidly correcting serum sodium with hypertonic saline in this setting makes the patients prone to more complications rather than the hyponatremia itself.

4. Vaptans

Vaptans are "vasopressin receptor antagonists" and have been studied, mainly in heart failure and in the setting of cirrhosis [38, 39]. Their value in treating hyponatremia and in reducing fluid overload has been investigated. They appear to be useful in treating mild hyponatremia. However, correction of hyponatremia solely may not associate with more important clinical outcomes. The intravenous agent conivaptan has been approved for use for treatment of euvolemic and hypervolemic hyponatremia in hospitalized patients [38]. The manufacturer advises clinician to exercise extra precaution as rapid correction of hyponatremia can have serious/irreversible clinical outcomes, i.e., central pontine myelinolysis. An oral formulation—tolvaptan—increases serum sodium in patients who have baseline values of <130 mmol/L [40]. Of note, correction of sodium is not permanent, and hyponatremia may return when medication is stopped [41].

Recently, satavaptan was particularly investigated to define its effectiveness in managing ascites rather than hyponatremia, was found to be "not clinically beneficial" in the controlling of ascites in cirrhosis, and was linked with higher mortality compared to placebo [42]. It is also more expensive than first-line therapy.

5. Intravenous albumin

An open-label, randomized controlled trial in patients with new onset ascites demonstrates that weekly 25 g infusions of albumin for 1 year followed by infusions every 2 weeks improved survival and decreased the risk of ascite recurrence compared to diuretics alone [43].

In patients who undergo large-volume paracentesis (LVP) > 5 L secondary to refractory ascites, the administration of albumin prevents post-paracentesis circulatory dysfunction (PPCD) [44]. Circulatory homeostasis has detrimental effects in cirrhotic patients as it leads to rapid re-buildup of ascites [45]. Around 20% of these patients develop dilutional hyponatremia secondary to hepatorenal syndrome and/or water retention. The portal pressure usually rises in patients developing circulatory dysfunction after LVP, probably due to a raised intrahepatic resistance due to the action of vasoconstrictor systems on the hepatic vascular bed [46–54]. Finally and most importantly, circulatory dysfunction is usually linked to decreased survival [44, 53].

LVP coupled with albumin infusion is more effective than diuretics and significantly cuts the length of hospital stay. It also has lower frequency of hyponatremia, renal impairment, and hepatic encephalopathy when compared with diuretics. However, there were no differences between the two approaches with respect to hospital readmission or survival [45, 55].

Albumin has shown to be more effective than dextran-70 and polygeline (other plasma expanders) for the stoppage of PPCD [44]. If <5 L of ascites are eliminated, dextran-70 (8 g/L of ascites removed) and polygeline (150 mL/L of ascites removed) show effectiveness comparable to that of albumin. Nevertheless, albumin has higher efficacy than these other plasma expanders if in the case of removal of more than 5 L of ascetic fluid [44]. In spite of that, randomized trials did not show survival advantage in patients treated with albumin versus those treated with other plasma expanders [44, 53, 56]. To demonstrate survival benefit of albumin, larger trials are warranted. Of note, a published meta-analysis included 17 trials involving 1225 patients, demonstrating a lessening in mortality with an odds ratio of death of 0.64 (95% CI, 0.41–0.98) in the albumin group [57, 58]. Albumin was superior to other plasma expanders in which a mean volume of ascetic fluid removed was 5.5–15.9 L [58]. Studies have administered between 5 and 10 g of albumin per liter of fluid removed; 6–8 g/L have been the most frequently used doses [58]. Another study compared albumin doses in 70 patients; the 4 g/L group had comparable PPCD and renal impairment to the 8 g/L group [46, 59].

Albumin is usually infused throughout and/or shortly after the paracentesis. In Europe, only a 20% intravenous solution is available. While in the United States, 5% and 25% intravenous solutions are available, all are isotonic. Using the 5% solution increases the sodium load five times.

6. Drugs to be avoided or used with caution

Angiotensin-converting enzyme inhibitors and angiotensin receptor blockers should be avoided in patients with cirrhosis and ascites even in low doses as they can induce arterial hypotension and renal failure [60, 61]. If used, blood pressure and renal function must be monitored carefully [7].

The administration of nonsteroidal anti-inflammatory drugs (NSAIDs), such as indomethacin, ibuprofen, and aspirin, in patients with cirrhosis and ascites is associated with a high risk of development of acute renal failure and hyponatremia and lowers the effect of diuretics [7]. This occurs primarily due to inhibition of renal prostaglandin synthesis leading to deficiency in glomerular filtration rate, which is due to a reduced renal perfusion [62]. Cyclooxygenase-2 (COX-2) inhibitors may provide an alternative for short term as preliminary data show that short-term administration of celecoxib does not impair renal function and does not alter response to diuretics [62].

Beta-blockers have been shown to reduce survival in patients with refractory ascites [63, 64]. This has been linked to their undesirable effect on blood pressure and the increase in the rate of paracentesis-induced circulatory dysfunction [63, 64].

Both blood pressure and renal function should be monitored closely in patients who have refractory ascites with consideration not to initiate or discontinue beta-blockers in such setting.

7. Colloid replacement

Colloid replacement therapy remains as a contentious issue in therapeutic paracentesis. One study compared the use of albumin (10 g/L of fluid removed) versus no albumin in 105 patients with tense ascites, following therapeutic paracentesis [65]. The no-albumin group had statistically significantly more changes in electrolytes, plasma renin, and serum creatinine, but no more clinical morbidity or mortality compared to the albumin group [65]. There are no studies that demonstrate decreased survival in patients without plasma expander compared to patients given with albumin after paracentesis [44].

Polygeline (plasma expander) is no longer used in many countries because of the possible risk of transmission of prions. Some evidence suggest that the use of saline is not linked to a high risk to develop PPCD after small-volume paracentesis [53]; there are no randomized controlled studies comparing saline versus albumin in patients who require paracentesis of less than 5 L. The use of starch as a plasma expander has been addressed in few studies in patients with cirrhosis and grade 3 ascites treated with LVP, revealing some concerning issues regarding the likelihood for starch to induce renal failure and hepatic accumulation of starch [66, 67].

On the other hand, a health economic analysis model suggested that it is more cost-effective to use albumin after LVP compared with alternative cheaper plasma volume expanders. This finding was mainly attributed to the fact that the administration of albumin post-paracentesis is associated with a smaller number of liver-related complications within the first 30 days which leads to increased total health cost [56].

8. Other treatment options

Activation of neurohumoral systems with sodium and water retention plays a major role in the pathogenesis of refractory ascites; thus, drugs that may improve circulatory and renal function, principally vasoconstrictors, have been investigated. Vasoconstrictors such as the $\alpha 1$-adrenergic agonist midodrine or terlipressin improve circulatory and renal function in patients with and without refractory ascites. Terlipressin is given in intravenous boluses (1 mg at onset of paracentesis, 1 mg at 8 h and 1 mg at 16 h) in addition to oral midodrine (for 72 h post-paracentesis), which appear to be as good as albumin in suppressing plasma renin elevation in randomized trials; terlipressin is not commercially offered in the United States [51, 68, 69].

9. Spontaneous bacterial peritonitis (SBP)

Ascitic fluid infection is common (12% in older series) and is associated with mortality rate that surpassed 90% [70–72]. This mortality rate can be reduced to 20% with early diagnosis and treatment [6, 73]. The diagnosis of spontaneous bacterial peritonitis (SBP) is made in the presence of raised ascitic fluid absolute polymorphonuclear leukocyte (PMN) count (i.e., ≥250 cells/mm^3 [0.25×10^9/L]). Treatment of SBP is a separate topic; we will discuss the importance of albumin and other therapies in addition to antibiotic use.

10. Empiric treatment

Empiric antibiotic therapy should be initiated in patients with ascitic fluid PMN counts greater than or equal to 250 cells/mm^3 (0.25×10^9/L). About 60% of the patients present with culture-negative ascites. If cultures are positive, however, the most common pathogens include Gram-negative bacteria (GNB), usually *Escherichia coli* and Gram-positive cocci (mainly streptococcus species and enterococci) [71, 74]. The epidemiology of bacterial infections differs between community-acquired (in which GNB infections predominate) and nosocomial infections (in which Gram-positive infections predominate).

Moderately broad-spectrum therapy is necessary in patients with suspected ascitic fluid infection unless otherwise indicated by culture and sensitivity when available. In a controlled trial, cefotaxime, a cephalosporin from the third generation, is shown to be superior to ampicillin plus tobramycin [75]. Cefotaxime or a similar third-generation cephalosporin seems to be the best therapeutic option for anticipated SBP; it is used to cover 95% of the flora including the three most common isolates: *E. coli, Klebsiella pneumoniae,* and *Streptococcus pneumoniae* [75]; usually, a 5-day treatment is as effective as 10 days in the treatment [76]. To achieve ascetic fluid levels that are 20-fold above the killing power after 1 dose of cefotaxime, 2 g intravenously every 8 h is required [77]. In neutrocytic ascites, a 5-day course of ceftriaxone 1 g intravenously twice per day was sufficient in treating culture-negative ascites [78].

Amoxicillin/clavulanic acid, intravenously and then orally, has comparable outcomes with respect to SBP resolution and mortality, compared with cefotaxime [79] and at reduced cost.

Another antibiotic that produces a similar SBP resolution rate and hospital survival compared with cefotaxime is ciprofloxacin. Ciprofloxacin is administered as either for 7 days intravenously or for 2 days intravenously followed by 5 days orally. Nevertheless, the cost is higher compared with cephalosporin-based options [80]. However, the use of intravenous antibiotic at the start, followed by oral step-down administration with ciprofloxacin, is more cost-effective than intravenous cefotaxime [81]. Ofloxacin also has produced similar results to intravenous cefotaxime when given orally in uncomplicated SBP, without renal failure, hepatic encephalopathy, gastrointestinal bleeding, ileus, or shock [82].

It is important to mention that, if ascitic fluid neutrophil count does not decrease to less than 25% of the pretreatment value after 48 h of antibiotic treatment, there is a high likelihood of failure to respond to therapy [83, 84]. In such scenarios antibiotic therapy should be broaden to cover more resistant pathogens.

11. Secondary prophylaxis of spontaneous bacterial peritonitis

The ideal prophylactic agent should be safe, affordable, and effective at decreasing the episodes of SBP while preserving the protective anaerobic flora (selective intestinal decontamination) [73]. Given the high cost and the risk of developing resistant organisms, the use of prophylactic antibiotics must be strictly restricted to patients with the following risk factors: (1) patients with acute gastrointestinal hemorrhage, (2) patients with low total protein content in ascitic fluid and no prior history of SBP (primary prophylaxis), and (3) patients with a previous history of SBP (secondary prophylaxis).

The cumulative recurrence rate at 1 year is approximately 70% in patients who survive an episode of SBP with survival rate of up to 30–50% and falls to 25–30% at 2 years [73]. Several antimicrobial regimens have been proposed as secondary prophylaxis. Norfloxacin was studied in a randomized, double-blind, placebo-controlled trial of (400 mg/day orally) in patients who had a previous episode of SBP [85, 86]. Norfloxacin was found to reduce the likelihood of SBP recurrence from 68 to 20% and the likelihood of SBP due to Gram-negative bacteria from 60 to 3%. Other studies evaluated the impact of ciprofloxacin, trimethoprim-sulfamethoxazole, and norfloxacin on SBP recurrence, but they included patients with and without previous episodes of SBP. All studies showed a reduced incidence of SBP with antibiotic prophylaxis [87–89].

The emergence of resistant, extended-spectrum B-lactamase-producing *Enterobacteriaceae* has occurred as a result of the extensive use of quinolones to prevent SBP [90–92].

Alternatively, ofloxacin, dosed at 400 mg bid for about 8 days, was found to be as good as parenteral cefotaxime in the treatment of SBP in patients without vomiting, shock, grade II (or higher) hepatic encephalopathy, or serum creatinine greater than 3 mg/dL [82]. A more cost-effective choice when compared to intravenous ceftazidime in a randomized trial would be the administration of intravenous ciprofloxacin followed by oral administration in patients who had not received quinolone prophylaxis [93]. Patients' flora may become resistant to quinolone prophylaxis, and hence treatment with alternative agents is warranted.

Reduction in mortality was reported in one trial when patients with SBP were randomized to receive cefotaxime alone versus cefotaxime plus 1.5 g albumin per kg body weight within 6 h of enrollment and 1.0 g/kg on day 3. A reduction in mortality from 29 to 10% was described [93]. Another study has revealed that albumin must be administered when the

http://dx.doi.org/10.5772/intechopen.70544

serum creatinine is >1 mg/dL, total bilirubin >4 mg/dL, or blood urea nitrogen >30 mg/dL. If the patient does not meet these prerequisite criteria, then albumin is not indicated [94–97]. Albumin is superior to hydroxyethyl starch in spontaneous bacterial peritonitis [98].

Author details

Aziza Ajlan[1], Waleed K. Al-hamoudi[2,3] and Hussein Elsiesy[2,4*]

*Address all correspondence to: helsiesy@gmail.com

1 Department of Pharmacy, King Faisal Specialist Hospital & Research Center, Riyadh, Saudi Arabia

2 Department of Liver Transplantation, King Faisal Specialist Hospital & Research Center, Riyadh, Saudi Arabia

3 Division of Gastroenterology, King Saud University, Riyadh, Saudi Arabia

4 Department of Medicine, Alfaisal University, Riyadh, Saudi Arabia

References

[1] Asrani SK, Larson JJ, Yawn B, Therneau TM, Kim WR. Underestimation of liver-related mortality in the United States. Gastroenterology. 2013;**145**(2):375-82 e1-2.

[2] Lucena MI, Andrade RJ, Tognoni G, Hidalgo R, De La Cuesta FS, Spanish Collaborative Study Group on Therapeutic Management in Liver D. Multicenter hospital study on prescribing patterns for prophylaxis and treatment of complications of cirrhosis. European Journal of Clinical Pharmacology. 2002;**58**(6):435-40.

[3] Ripoll C, Groszmann R, Garcia-Tsao G, Grace N, Burroughs A, Planas R, et al. Hepatic venous pressure gradient predicts clinical decompensation in patients with compensated cirrhosis. Gastroenterology. 2007;**133**(2):481-88.

[4] Schrier RW, Arroyo V, Bernardi M, Epstein M, Henriksen JH, Rodes J. Peripheral arterial vasodilation hypothesis: A proposal for the initiation of renal sodium and water retention in cirrhosis. Hepatology. 1988;**8**(5):1151-7.

[5] Schomerus H, Heinrich R. Systemic manifestations of liver cirrhosis. Heart, circulation, lung. Zeitschrift für Gastroenterologie. Verhandlungsband. 1986;**21**:21-6.

[6] Tandon P, Garcia-Tsao G. Bacterial infections, sepsis, and multiorgan failure in cirrhosis. Seminars in Liver Disease. 2008;**28**(1):26-42.

[7] European Association for the Study of the L. EASL clinical practice guidelines on the management of ascites, spontaneous bacterial peritonitis, and hepatorenal syndrome in cirrhosis. Journal of Hepatology. 2010;**53**(3):397-417.

[8] BA R. Sleisenger and Fordtran's Gastrointestinal and Liver Disease. Philadelphia: Saunders Elsevier; 2010. pp. 1517-41.

[9] Veldt BJ, Laine F, Guillygomarc'h A, Lauvin L, Boudjema K, Messner M, et al. Indication of liver transplantation in severe alcoholic liver cirrhosis: Quantitative evaluation and optimal timing. Journal of Hepatology. 2002;**36**(1):93-98.

[10] Garg H, Sarin SK, Kumar M, Garg V, Sharma BC, Kumar A. Tenofovir improves the outcome in patients with spontaneous reactivation of hepatitis B presenting as acute-on-chronic liver failure. Hepatology. 2011;**53**(3):774-80.

[11] Montero E, Miguel J, Lopez-Alvarez J. Care of patients with ascites. The New England Journal of Medicine. 1994;**330**(25):1828.

[12] Angeli P, Gatta A, Caregaro L, Menon F, Sacerdoti D, Merkel C, et al. Tubular site of renal sodium retention in ascitic liver cirrhosis evaluated by lithium clearance. European Journal of Clinical Investigation. 1990;**20**(1):111-7.

[13] Angeli P, De Bei E, Dalla Pria M, Caregaro L, Ceolotto G, Albino G, et al. Effects of amiloride on renal lithium handling in nonazotemic ascitic cirrhotic patients with avid sodium retention. Hepatology. 1992;**15**(4):651-4.

[14] Bernardi M, Servadei D, Trevisani F, Rusticali AG, Gasbarrini G. Importance of plasma aldosterone concentration on the natriuretic effect of spironolactone in patients with liver cirrhosis and ascites. Digestion. 1985;**31**(4):189-93.

[15] Angeli P, Dalla Pria M, De Bei E, Albino G, Caregaro L, Merkel C, et al. Randomized clinical study of the efficacy of amiloride and potassium canrenoate in nonazotemic cirrhotic patients with ascites. Hepatology. 1994;**19**(1):72-9.

[16] Angeli P, Fasolato S, Mazza E, Okolicsanyi L, Maresio G, Velo E, et al. Combined versus sequential diuretic treatment of ascites in non-azotaemic patients with cirrhosis: Results of an open randomised clinical trial. Gut. 2010;**59**(1):98-104.

[17] Santos J, Planas R, Pardo A, Durandez R, Cabre E, Morillas RM, et al. Spironolactone alone or in combination with furosemide in the treatment of moderate ascites in nonazotemic cirrhosis. A randomized comparative study of efficacy and safety. Journal of Hepatology. 2003;**39**(2):187-92.

[18] Pitt B, Remme W, Zannad F, Neaton J, Martinez F, Roniker B, et al. Eplerenone, a selective aldosterone blocker, in patients with left ventricular dysfunction after myocardial infarction. The New England Journal of Medicine. 2003;**348**(14):1309-21.

[19] Singh HJ, Singh S, Chander R, Charan S. Comparative study of spironolactone and eplerenone in management of ascites in cirrhosis liver. The Journal of the Association of Physicians of India. 2016;**64**(1):48.

[20] Mimidis K, Papadopoulos V, Kartalis G. Eplerenone relieves spironolactone-induced painful gynaecomastia in patients with decompensated hepatitis B-related cirrhosis. Scandinavian Journal of Gastroenterology. 2007;**42**(12):1516-7.

[21] Elfert AA, Abo Ali L, Soliman S, Zakaria S, Shehab El-Din I, Elkhalawany W, et al. Randomized placebo-controlled study of baclofen in the treatment of muscle cramps in patients with liver cirrhosis. European Journal of Gastroenterology & Hepatology. 2016;**28**(11):1280-4.

[22] Chatrath H, Liangpunsakul S, Ghabril M, Otte J, Chalasani N, Vuppalanchi R. Prevalence and morbidity associated with muscle cramps in patients with cirrhosis. The American Journal of Medicine. 2012;**125**(10):1019-25.

[23] Atluri DK, Veluru C, Mullen K. An alternative treatment for muscle cramps in patients with liver cirrhosis. Liver International: Official Journal of the International Association for the Study of the Liver. 2013;**33**(3):496-7.

[24] Henry ZH, Northup PG. Baclofen for the treatment of muscle cramps in patients with cirrhosis: A new alternative. Hepatology. 2016;**64**(2):695-6.

[25] Angeli P, Albino G, Carraro P, Dalla Pria M, Merkel C, Caregaro L, et al. Cirrhosis and muscle cramps: Evidence of a causal relationship. Hepatology. 1996;**23**(2):264-73.

[26] Nakanishi H, Kurosaki M, Tsuchiya K, Nakakuki N, Takada H, Matsuda S, et al. L-carnitine reduces muscle cramps in patients with cirrhosis. Clinical Gastroenterology and Hepatology. 2015;**13**(8):1540-3.

[27] Mehta SS, Fallon MB. Muscle cramps in cirrhosis: A moving target. Clinical Gastroenterology and Hepatology. 2015;**13**(8):1544-6.

[28] Corbani A, Manousou P, Calvaruso V, Xirouchakis I, Burroughs AK. Muscle cramps in cirrhosis: The therapeutic value of quinine. Is it underused? Digestive and Liver Disease: Official Journal of the Italian Society of Gastroenterology and the Italian Association for the Study of the Liver. 2008;**40**(9):794-9.

[29] Abrams GA, Concato J, Fallon MB. Muscle cramps in patients with cirrhosis. The American Journal of Gastroenterology. 1996;**91**(7):1363-6.

[30] Marotta PJ, Graziadei IW, Ghent CN. Muscle cramps: A 'complication' of cirrhosis. Canadian Journal of Gastroenterology. 2000;**14**(Suppl D):21D-5D.

[31] Marchesini G, Bianchi G, Amodio P, Salerno F, Merli M, Panella C, et al. Factors associated with poor health-related quality of life of patients with cirrhosis. Gastroenterology. 2001;**120**(1):170-8.

[32] Qavi AH, Kamal R, Schrier RW. Clinical use of diuretics in heart failure, cirrhosis, and nephrotic syndrome. International Journal of Nephrology. 2015;**2015**:975934.

[33] Knauf H, Mutschler E. Liver cirrhosis with ascites: Pathogenesis of resistance to diuretics and long-term efficacy and safety of torasemide. Cardiology. 1994;**84**(Suppl 2):87-98.

[34] Porayko MK, Wiesner RH. Management of ascites in patients with cirrhosis. What to do when diuretics fail. Postgraduate Medicine. 1992;**92**(8):155-158 61-6.

[35] Bernardi M. Optimum use of diuretics in managing ascites in patients with cirrhosis. Gut. 2010;**59**(1):10-1.

[36] Planas R, Pardo A, Durandez R, Cabre E, Morillas RM, Granada ML, et al. Spironolactone alone or in combination with furosemide in the treatment of moderate ascites in non-azotemic cirrhosis. A randomized comparative study of efficacy and safety. Journal of Hepatology. 2003;**39**(2):187-92.

[37] Vidot H, Carey S, Allman-Farinelli M, Shackel N. Systematic review: The treatment of muscle cramps in patients with cirrhosis. Alimentary Pharmacology & Therapeutics. 2014;**40**(3): 221-32.

[38] Wong F, Blei AT, Blendis LM, Thuluvath PJ. A vasopressin receptor antagonist (VPA-985) improves serum sodium concentration in patients with hyponatremia: A multi-center, randomized, placebo-controlled trial. Hepatology. 2003;**37**(1):182-191.

[39] Schrier RW, Gross P, Gheorghiade M, Berl T, Verbalis JG, Czerwiec FS, et al. Tolvaptan, a selective oral vasopressin V2-receptor antagonist, for hyponatremia. The New England Journal of Medicine. 2006;**355**(20):2099-2112.

[40] Yamada T, Ohki T, Hayata Y, Karasawa Y, Kawamura S, Ito D, et al. Potential effectiveness of tolvaptan to improve ascites unresponsive to standard diuretics and overall survival in patients with decompensated liver cirrhosis. Clinical Drug Investigation. 2016;**36**(10):829-35.

[41] Cardenas A, Gines P, Marotta P, Czerwiec F, Oyuang J, Guevara M, et al. Tolvaptan, an oral vasopressin antagonist, in the treatment of hyponatremia in cirrhosis. Journal of Hepatology. 2012;**56**(3):571-8.

[42] Wong F, Watson H, Gerbes A, Vilstrup H, Badalamenti S, Bernardi M, et al. Satavaptan for the management of ascites in cirrhosis: Efficacy and safety across the spectrum of ascites severity. Gut. 2012;**61**(1):108-16.

[43] Romanelli RG, La Villa G, Barletta G, Vizzutti F, Lanini F, Arena U, et al. Long-term albumin infusion improves survival in patients with cirrhosis and ascites: An unblinded randomized trial. World Journal of Gastroenterology. 2006;**12**(9):1403-7.

[44] Gines A, Fernandez-Esparrach G, Monescillo A, Vila C, Domenech E, Abecasis R, et al. Randomized trial comparing albumin, dextran 70, and polygeline in cirrhotic patients with ascites treated by paracentesis. Gastroenterology. 1996;**111**(4):1002-10.

[45] Sola R, Vila MC, Andreu M, Oliver MI, Coll S, Gana J, et al. Total paracentesis with dextran 40 vs diuretics in the treatment of ascites in cirrhosis: A randomized controlled study. Journal of Hepatology. 1994;**20**(2):282-8.

[46] Hoefs JC. Prevention of the paracentesis-induced circulatory dysfunction (PICD) in cirrhosis: Is the SPA treatment worthwhile? Digestive Diseases and Sciences. 2016;**61**(10):2773-5.

[47] Tan HK, James PD, Wong F. Albumin may prevent the morbidity of Paracentesis-induced circulatory dysfunction in cirrhosis and refractory ascites: A pilot study. Digestive Diseases and Sciences. 2016;**61**(10):3084-92.

[48] Kim JH. What we know about paracentesis induced circulatory dysfunction? Clinical and Molecular Hepatology. 2015;**21**(4):349-51.

[49] Bai M, Han G. Midodrine for paracentesis-induced circulatory dysfunction. Journal of Clinical Gastroenterology. 2014;**48**(3):300.

[50] Hamdy H, ElBaz AA, Hassan A, Hassanin O. Comparison of midodrine and albumin in the prevention of paracentesis-induced circulatory dysfunction in cirrhotic patients: A randomized pilot study. Journal of Clinical Gastroenterology. 2014;**48**(2):184-8.

[51] Singh V, Dheerendra PC, Singh B, Nain CK, Chawla D, Sharma N, et al. Midodrine versus albumin in the prevention of paracentesis-induced circulatory dysfunction in cirrhotics: A randomized pilot study. The American Journal of Gastroenterology. 2008;**103**(6):1399-405.

[52] Appenrodt B, Wolf A, Grunhage F, Trebicka J, Schepke M, Rabe C, et al. Prevention of paracentesis-induced circulatory dysfunction: Midodrine vs albumin. A randomized pilot study. Liver International: Official Journal of the International Association for the Study of the Liver. 2008;**28**(7):1019-25.

[53] Sola-Vera J, Minana J, Ricart E, Planella M, Gonzalez B, Torras X, et al. Randomized trial comparing albumin and saline in the prevention of paracentesis-induced circulatory dysfunction in cirrhotic patients with ascites. Hepatology. 2003;**37**(5):1147-53.

[54] Ruiz-del-Arbol L, Monescillo A, Jimenez W, Garcia-Plaza A, Arroyo V, Rodes J. Paracentesis-induced circulatory dysfunction: Mechanism and effect on hepatic hemodynamics in cirrhosis. Gastroenterology. 1997;**113**(2):579-86.

[55] Acharya SK, Balwinder S, Padhee AK, Nijhawan S, Tandon BN. Large volume paracentesis and intravenous dextran to treat tense ascites. Journal of Clinical Gastroenterology. 1992;**14**(1):31-5.

[56] Moreau R, Valla DC, Durand-Zaleski I, Bronowicki JP, Durand F, Chaput JC, et al. Comparison of outcome in patients with cirrhosis and ascites following treatment with albumin or a synthetic colloid: A randomised controlled pilot trail. Liver International: Official Journal of the International Association for the Study of the Liver. 2006;**26**(1):46-54.

[57] Bernardi M, Caraceni P, Navickis RJ. Does the evidence support a survival benefit of albumin infusion in patients with cirrhosis undergoing large-volume paracentesis? Expert Review of Gastroenterology & Hepatology. 2017;**11**(3):191-192.

[58] Bernardi M, Caraceni P, Navickis RJ, Wilkes MM. Albumin infusion in patients undergoing large-volume paracentesis: A meta-analysis of randomized trials. Hepatology. 2012;**55**(4):1172-81.

[59] Alessandria C, Elia C, Mezzabotta L, Risso A, Andrealli A, Spandre M, et al. Prevention of paracentesis-induced circulatory dysfunction in cirrhosis: Standard vs half albumin doses. A prospective, randomized, unblinded pilot study. Digestive and Liver Disease: Official Journal of the Italian Society of Gastroenterology and the Italian Association for the Study of the Liver. 2011;**43**(11):881-6.

[60] Pariente EA, Bataille C, Bercoff E, Lebrec D. Acute effects of captopril on systemic and renal hemodynamics and on renal function in cirrhotic patients with ascites. Gastroenterology. 1985;**88**(5 Pt 1):1255-9.

[61] Gentilini P, Romanelli RG, La Villa G, Maggiore Q, Pesciullesi E, Cappelli G, et al. Effects of low-dose captopril on renal hemodynamics and function in patients with cirrhosis of the liver. Gastroenterology. 1993;**104**(2):588-94.

[62] Claria J, Kent JD, Lopez-Parra M, Escolar G, Ruiz-Del-Arbol L, Gines P, et al. Effects of celecoxib and naproxen on renal function in nonazotemic patients with cirrhosis and ascites. Hepatology. 2005;**41**(3):579-87.

[63] Kurt M. Deleterious effects of beta-blockers on survival in patients with cirrhosis and refractory ascites. Hepatology. 2011;**53**(4):1411-2.

[64] Serste T, Melot C, Francoz C, Durand F, Rautou PE, Valla D, et al. Deleterious effects of beta-blockers on survival in patients with cirrhosis and refractory ascites. Hepatology. 2010;**52**(3): 1017-22.

[65] Gines P, Tito L, Arroyo V, Planas R, Panes J, Viver J, et al. Randomized comparative study of therapeutic paracentesis with and without intravenous albumin in cirrhosis. Gastroenterology. 1988;**94**(6):1493-502.

[66] Brunkhorst FM, Engel C, Bloos F, Meier-Hellmann A, Ragaller M, Weiler N, et al. Intensive insulin therapy and pentastarch resuscitation in severe sepsis. The New England Journal of Medicine. 2008;**358**(2):125-39.

[67] Christidis C, Mal F, Ramos J, Senejoux A, Callard P, Navarro R, et al. Worsening of hepatic dysfunction as a consequence of repeated hydroxyethylstarch infusions. Journal of Hepatology. 2001;**35**(6):726-32.

[68] Angeli P, Volpin R, Piovan D, Bortoluzzi A, Craighero R, Bottaro S, et al. Acute effects of the oral administration of midodrine, an alpha-adrenergic agonist, on renal hemodynamics and renal function in cirrhotic patients with ascites. Hepatology. 1998;**28**(4):937-43.

[69] Krag A, Moller S, Henriksen JH, Holstein-Rathlou NH, Larsen FS, Bendtsen F. Terlipressin improves renal function in patients with cirrhosis and ascites without hepatorenal syndrome. Hepatology. 2007;**46**(6):1863-71.

[70] Zhang JM, Weng XH. Diagnosis, treatment and prophylaxis of spontaneous bacterial peritonitis. Zhonghua Gan Zang Bing Za Zhi. 2005;**13**(6):459-60.

[71] Rimola A, Garcia-Tsao G, Navasa M, Piddock LJ, Planas R, Bernard B, et al. Diagnosis, treatment and prophylaxis of spontaneous bacterial peritonitis: A consensus document. International ascites Club. Journal of Hepatology. 2000;**32**(1):142-53.

[72] Navasa M, Casafont F, Clemente G, Guarner C, de la Mata M, Planas R, et al. Consensus on spontaneous bacterial peritonitis in liver cirrhosis: Diagnosis, treatment, and prophylaxis. Gastroenterología y Hepatología. 2001;**24**(1):37-46.

[73] Garcia-Tsao G. Current Management of the Complications of cirrhosis and portal hypertension: Variceal hemorrhage, ascites, and spontaneous bacterial peritonitis. Digestive Diseases. 2016;**34**(4):382-6.

[74] Fernandez J, Navasa M, Gomez J, Colmenero J, Vila J, Arroyo V, et al. Bacterial infections in cirrhosis: Epidemiological changes with invasive procedures and norfloxacin prophylaxis. Hepatology. 2002;**35**(1):140-8.

[75] Felisart J, Rimola A, Arroyo V, Perez-Ayuso RM, Quintero E, Gines P, et al. Cefotaxime is more effective than is ampicillin-tobramycin in cirrhotics with severe infections. Hepatology. 1985;**5**(3):457-62.

[76] Runyon BA, McHutchison JG, Antillon MR, Akriviadis EA, Montano AA. Short-course versus long-course antibiotic treatment of spontaneous bacterial peritonitis. A randomized controlled study of 100 patients. Gastroenterology. 1991;**100**(6):1737-42.

[77] Runyon BA, Akriviadis EA, Sattler FR, Cohen J. Ascitic fluid and serum cefotaxime and desacetyl cefotaxime levels in patients treated for bacterial peritonitis. Digestive Diseases and Sciences. 1991;**36**(12):1782-6.

[78] Baskol M, Gursoy S, Baskol G, Ozbakir O, Guven K, Yucesoy M. Five days of ceftriaxone to treat culture negative neutrocytic ascites in cirrhotic patients. Journal of Clinical Gastroenterology. 2003;**37**(5):403-5.

[79] Ricart E, Soriano G, Novella MT, Ortiz J, Sabat M, Kolle L, et al. Amoxicillin-clavulanic acid versus cefotaxime in the therapy of bacterial infections in cirrhotic patients. Journal of Hepatology. 2000;**32**(4):596-602.

[80] Terg R, Cobas S, Fassio E, Landeira G, Rios B, Vasen W, et al. Oral ciprofloxacin after a short course of intravenous ciprofloxacin in the treatment of spontaneous bacterial peritonitis: Results of a multicenter, randomized study. Journal of Hepatology. 2000;**33**(4):564-9.

[81] Angeli P, Guarda S, Fasolato S, Miola E, Craighero R, Piccolo F, et al. Switch therapy with ciprofloxacin vs. intravenous ceftazidime in the treatment of spontaneous bacterial peritonitis in patients with cirrhosis: Similar efficacy at lower cost. Alimentary Pharmacology & Therapeutics. 2006;**23**(1):75-84.

[82] Navasa M, Follo A, Llovet JM, Clemente G, Vargas V, Rimola A, et al. Randomized, comparative study of oral ofloxacin versus intravenous cefotaxime in spontaneous bacterial peritonitis. Gastroenterology. 1996;**111**(4):1011-7.

[83] Guarner C, Soriano G. Spontaneous bacterial peritonitis. Seminars in Liver Disease. 1997; **17**(3):203-17.

[84] Brahmbhatt R, Tapper EB. Optimizing the outcomes associated with spontaneous bacterial peritonitis. Journal of Clinical Gastroenterology. 2017;**51**(3):191-4.

[85] Gines P, Rimola A, Planas R, Vargas V, Marco F, Almela M, et al. Norfloxacin prevents spontaneous bacterial peritonitis recurrence in cirrhosis: Results of a double-blind, placebo-controlled trial. Hepatology. 1990;**12**(4 Pt 1):716-24.

[86] Bauer TM, Follo A, Navasa M, Vila J, Planas R, Clemente G, et al. Daily norfloxacin is more effective than weekly rufloxacin in prevention of spontaneous bacterial peritonitis recurrence. Digestive Diseases and Sciences. 2002;**47**(6):1356-61.

[87] Soriano G, Guarner C, Teixido M, Such J, Barrios J, Enriquez J, et al. Selective intestinal decontamination prevents spontaneous bacterial peritonitis. Gastroenterology. 1991;**100**(2): 477-81.

[88] Rolachon A, Cordier L, Bacq Y, Nousbaum JB, Franza A, Paris JC, et al. Ciprofloxacin and long-term prevention of spontaneous bacterial peritonitis: Results of a prospective controlled trial. Hepatology. 1995;**22**(4 Pt 1):1171-4.

[89] Singh N, Gayowski T, Yu VL, Wagener MM. Trimethoprim-sulfamethoxazole for the prevention of spontaneous bacterial peritonitis in cirrhosis: A randomized trial. Annals of Internal Medicine. 1995;**122**(8):595-8.

[90] Fernandez J, Acevedo J, Castro M, Garcia O, de Lope CR, Roca D, et al. Prevalence and risk factors of infections by multiresistant bacteria in cirrhosis: A prospective study. Hepatology. 2012;**55**(5):1551-61.

[91] Ariza X, Castellote J, Lora-Tamayo J, Girbau A, Salord S, Rota R, et al. Risk factors for resistance to ceftriaxone and its impact on mortality in community, healthcare and nosocomial spontaneous bacterial peritonitis. Journal of Hepatology. 2012;**56**(4):825-32.

[92] Runyon BA. Changing Flora of bacterial infections in patients with cirrhosis. Liver International : Official Journal of the International Association for the Study of the Liver. 2010;**30**(9):1245-6.

[93] Sort P, Navasa M, Arroyo V, Aldeguer X, Planas R, Ruiz-del-Arbol L, et al. Effect of intravenous albumin on renal impairment and mortality in patients with cirrhosis and spontaneous bacterial peritonitis. The New England Journal of Medicine. 1999;**341**(6):403-9.

[94] Verma A, Lalchandani A, Giri R, Agarwal S, Priyadarshi BP. Evaluation of relation between spontaneous bacterial peritonitis and serum ascites albumin gradient as a prognostic risk factor in chronic liver disease. The Journal of the Association of Physicians of India. 2016;**64**(1):48.

[95] Jamtgaard L, Manning SL, Cohn B. Does albumin infusion reduce renal impairment and mortality in patients with spontaneous bacterial peritonitis? Annals of Emergency Medicine. 2016;**67**(4):458-9.

[96] Salerno F, Navickis RJ, Wilkes MM. Albumin infusion improves outcomes of patients with spontaneous bacterial peritonitis: A meta-analysis of randomized trials. Clinical Gastroenterology and Hepatology. 2013;**11**(2):123-30 e1.

[97] Sigal SH, Stanca CM, Fernandez J, Arroyo V, Navasa M. Restricted use of albumin for spontaneous bacterial peritonitis. Gut. 2007;**56**(4):597-9.

[98] Grange JD, Amiot X. Effect of intravenous albumin on renal impairment and mortality in patients with cirrhosis and spontaneous bacterial peritonitis. Gastroentérologie Clinique et Biologique. 2000;**24**(3):378-9.

Chapter 7

Predictors of the Response to Tolvaptan Therapy and Its Effect on Prognosis in Cirrhotic Patients with Ascites

Tomomi Kogiso, Kuniko Yamamoto,
Mutsuki Kobayashi, Yuichi Ikarashi,
Kazuhisa Kodama, Makiko Taniai, Nobuyuki Torii,
Etsuko Hashimoto and Katsutoshi Tokushige

Additional information is available at the end of the chapter

http://dx.doi.org/10.5772/intechopen.69849

Abstract

Aims: The vasopressin V2 receptor antagonist, tolvaptan, has been reported to be effective in cirrhotic patients with ascites. Here, we evaluated predictors of the response to tolvaptan. *Methods*: A total of 97 patients with cirrhosis (60 males; median age, 63 years) who had been treated for ascites with oral tolvaptan were enrolled. Tolvaptan efficacy was defined as urine volume increase of ≥500 mL or a urine volume ≥2000 mL/day on the day following treatment. Normalization of the serum sodium (Na) level after 1 week of treatment and the posttreatment survival rate was analyzed. *Results*: Tolvaptan therapy resulted in effective urination in 67% of patients. A multivariate analysis revealed that the blood urea nitrogen/creatinine (BUN/Cr) ratio and urinary Na/potassium (Na/K) ratio were predictive of the tolvaptan response ($p < 0.05$). The serum Na level was 135 (121–145) mEq/L, and normal levels were recovered in 50.0% of the patients with an initial Na level of <135 mEq/L. The posttreatment survival rate was significantly higher in patients who responded to tolvaptan therapy ($p < 0.05$). *Conclusions*: The combination of the initial BUN/Cr and urine Na/K ratios and a normalized serum Na level after 1 week was predictive of a favorable outcome to tolvaptan therapy.

Keywords: vasopressin V2 receptor antagonist, tolvaptan, blood urea nitrogen/creatinine ratio, urine sodium/potassium ratio, serum sodium

1. Introduction

Ascites accumulation is commonly observed in decompensated liver cirrhosis [1]. The symptoms of ascites lead to a poor quality of life and prognosis [2]. Recently, the vasopressin V2 receptor antagonist tolvaptan has been used for ascites treatment of cirrhosis in addition to spironolactone ± furosemide [3, 4]. The Japanese Society of Gastroenterology published evidence-based clinical practice guidelines in 2015 [5]. Tolvaptan is recommended for use before ascites drainage or administration of albumin because of its high efficacy irrespective of the serum albumin level [6]. While the serum sodium (Na) level is low in cirrhosis, it is increased in tolvaptan-treated patients because of free water clearance without accompanying Na elimination. In contrast, conventional diuretics promote hyponatremia and impair renal function. Thus, tolvaptan has benefits for the treatment of cirrhosis.

The mechanism underlying refractory ascites caused by liver cirrhosis has been hypothesized as one or more of the following [7, 8]: (1) hypo-osmotic pressure due to hypoalbuminemia; (2) a response to mesenteric and systemic vasodilation, accompanied by development of portal hypertension, which decreases the effective circulatory volume and depletes renal flow, leading to increased arginine vasopressin (AVP) release; increased AVP results in an increase in renin-angiotensin-aldosterone system activity; and (3) postsinusoidal obstruction and lymphatic edema. These multiple causative factors are associated with ascites accumulation.

Approximately 70% of tolvaptan-treated patients exhibit increased urination and achieve a reduction in body weight within 7–14 days [9, 10]. In addition to this short-term efficacy, tolvaptan also exerts long-term effects [11]. However, factors that predict the response to tolvaptan and its effect on prognosis are unclear. In this study, we focused on predictors of the tolvaptan response and the outcome of tolvaptan therapy.

2. Patients and methods

2.1. Patients

This was a single-center, retrospective observational study performed between September 2013 and March 2016. We enrolled a total of 97 Japanese cirrhotic patients (60 males, 62%) who received tolvaptan 3.75–7.5 mg/day (Samsca™; Otsuka Pharmaceutical Co. Ltd., Tokyo, Japan) after hospitalization for ascites treatment. They were treated with conventional diuretics.

2.2. Method

The patients were classified as responders or nonresponders to tolvaptan therapy. Tolvaptan efficacy was defined as a urine volume increase of ≥500 mL or a urine volume ≥2000 mL/day on the day following tolvaptan treatment, as described by Ohki et al. with slight modifications [12]. The baseline characteristics of patients, including age, sex, medications, and laboratory parameters, were evaluated. We investigated the changes in body weight and the serum Na level after 1 week of treatment and evaluated laboratory parameters. Tolvaptan was not used in patients with severe renal dysfunction (estimated glomerular filtration rate <15 mL/min/1.73 m^2 or a serum creatinine [Cr] level >3.5 mg/dL) or a hepatic coma scale score >II.

This study was conducted according to the principles of the Declaration of Helsinki, and the Institutional Review Board of Tokyo Women's Medical University Hospital (Tokyo, Japan) approved the study protocol (no. 3258-R). The results of this study, including figures and tables, were published in Hepatology Research [13] and were transferred with permission.

2.3. Statistical analysis

Data are presented as medians with minimum and maximum values. Significant differences between the two groups were assessed using the Mann–Whitney U-test and χ^2 test. The Statistical Package for the Social Sciences software (SPSS Institute, 11.01.J, Chicago, IL, USA) was used for the statistical analyses. Statistical significance was considered at $p < 0.05$.

3. Results

3.1. Response to tolvaptan according to urination and body weight parameters

The median age of the 97 patients (62% male) receiving tolvaptan treatment was 63 years (range, 22–90 years; **Table 1**). The underlying liver diseases and frequency of other ascites treatments did not differ significantly. The median increase in urine volume on the day after treatment was 690 mL (range: −530 to +3490 mL), while the median urine volume was 1675 mL/day (range: 195–6630 mL/day). The distributions of urination and body weight changes and their correlations with the tolvaptan response are shown in **Figure 1(a)**. The change in body weight after 1 week of treatment was −1.5 kg (−17.2 to +6.2 kg). A total urine volume ≥2000 mL was achieved in 40% of cases and an increase in the urine volume in ~50% of cases (**Figure 1b**). Approximately 40% of cases achieved a ≥2.0 kg body weight reduction after 1 week of treatment. Overall, 67% of the cases achieved the desired level of urination. In cases who responded to tolvaptan, the platelet count, urine Na level, and urine Na/potassium (K) ratio were higher, and the blood urea nitrogen (BUN)/Cr ratio was lower (**Table 2**). The serum Na level was 135 (121–145) mEq/L, and 39.2% of cases had an Na level of <135 mEq/L.

3.2. Urination-based predictors of the response to tolvaptan

Multivariate analysis revealed that the BUN/Cr ratio (odds ratio [OR], 1.08; 95% confidence interval [CI], 1.006–1.174; $p < 0.05$) and urine Na/K ratio (OR, 0.59; 95% CI, 0.366–0.855; $p < 0.01$) were predictors of the tolvaptan response (**Table 3**). In particular, patients who satisfied both

	Total (n = 97)	Responder (n = 65)	Nonresponder (n = 32)	p-value
Age (years)	63 (22–90)	62 (22–90)	63 (37–84)	0.21
Sex (% of males)	62	66	53	0.21
Underlying hepatitis (%) (viral/metabolic/PBC)	37/39/9	32/43/11	47/31/6	0.29
Complication (%) (varices/HCC/hepatic encephalopathy)	67/35/23	71/35/18	59/34/31	0.37
Diuretics				
Furosemide dose (mg/day)	20 (0–160)	20 (0–160)	20 (0–80)	0.96
Spironolactone dose (mg/day)	50 (0–400)	50 (0–400)	50 (0–400)	0.97
BCAA (%)	90	89	91	0.11
Administration of albumin (%)	62	63	59	0.65
CART or drainage (%)	41	38	47	0.43
Prognosis; death or transplantation (%)	45	37	63	0.03

Notes: PBC, primary biliary cholangitis; HCC, hepatocellular carcinoma; BCAA, branched-chain amino acid; CART, cell-free and concentrated ascites reinfusion therapy.

Table 1. Baseline characteristics of the patients.

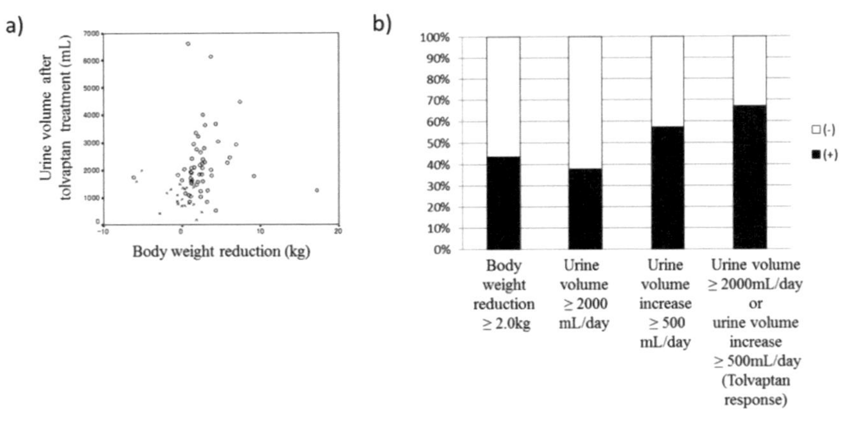

Figure 1. Urine volume and body weight response after tolvaptan treatment. (a) Distributions of urine volume after 1 day, and change in body weight after 1 week, of tolvaptan treatment. Circle, responder; cross, nonresponder. (b) The percentage of urination and body weight reduction responded to a tolvaptan therapy. Urine volume 1 day after, and change in body weight 1 week after, tolvaptan treatment was correlated with the tolvaptan response (a). A body weight reduction of ≥2.0 kg was found in 40% of cases, and a urine volume ≥2000 mL and a urine volume increase ≥500 mL were found in 67% of patients in response to tolvaptan therapy (b).

	Total (n = 97)	Responder (n = 65)	Nonresponder (n = 32)	p value
Albumin (g/dL)	2.5 (1.5–4.2)	2.5 (1.5–4.2)	2.4 (1.9–3.5)	0.88
Total bilirubin (mg/dL)	1.8 (0.3–52.4)	1.5 (0.5–33.0)	2.2 (0.3–52.4)	0.73
Platelet count ($\times 10^4$ μL^{-1})	8.6 (1.5–42.4)	9.0 (1.5–42.4)	6.4 (2.1–23.9)	0.05
Prothrombin time (%)	54.5 (16.3–90.3)	54.5 (16.3–90.3)	52.6 (22.6–89.0)	0.70
Ammonia (mg/dL)	69 (25–269)	70 (25–269)	63 (29–212)	0.97
α-Fetoprotein (ng/mL)	4 (1–29,292)	4 (1–4510)	6.5 (1–29,292)	0.36
DCP (mAU/mL)	75 (3–4994)	42 (3–4994)	324 (10–1788)	0.61
BUN (mg/dL)	23.4 (5.5–125.3)	21 (5.5–63.3)	27 (12.0–125.3)	0.02
Creatinine (mg/dL)	1.07 (0.20–3.30)	1.00 (0.42–2.12)	1.17 (0.50–3.30)	0.13
eGFR (mL/min/1.73 m^2)	50.0 (15.0–250.6)	50.3 (18–250.6)	46.2 (15.0–108.6)	0.15
Serum Na (mEq/L)	135 (121–145)	136 (122–145)	133 (121–144)	0.06
Serum K (mEq/L)	4.2 (2.8–6.1)	3.9 (2.8–5.3)	4.3 (3.1–6.1)	0.06
Serum osmolarity (mOsm/L)	281 (100–317)	283 (100–317)	279 (256–299)	0.68
Urine osmolarity (mOsm/L)	404 (116–938)	405 (116–938)	388 (233–715)	0.63
Urinary Na (mEq/L)	61 (7–256)	69.5 (10–256)	39 (7–108)	<0.01
Urinary K (mEq/L)	21 (6–72)	20 (6–72)	22 (13–48)	0.72
24 h creatinine clearance (mL/min)	51.2 (7.6–124.0)	52.8 (12.4–124.0)	44.1 (7.6–92.9)	0.12
BUN/creatinine ratio	22.5 (6.83–138.5)	21 (5.5–138.5)	23.7 (14.4–48.3)	0.01
Urine Na/K ratio	2.53 (0.22–25.6)	3.31 (0.35–25.6)	2.01 (0.22–5.13)	<0.01
Child-pugh score	10 (7–14)	10 (7–13)	10 (8–14)	0.23
Model for end-stage liver disease score	14 (7–31)	14 (7–31)	16 (8–31)	0.37

Notes. DCP; des-γ-carboxy prothrombin, BUN; blood urea nitrogen; eGFR, estimated glomerular filtration rate; Na/K; sodium/potassium.

Table 2. Laboratory data at initiation of tolvaptan treatment.

Parameter	Odds ratio	95% confidence interval	p-value
BUN/Cr ratio	1.08	1.006–1.174	<0.05
Urine Na/K ratio	0.59	0.366–0.855	<0.01
Serum K	1.41	0.537–3.893	n.s
Serum Na	0.96	0.854–1.080	n.s
Platelet count	0.95	0.839–1.051	n.s

Notes. Na/K, sodium/potassium; n.s, not significant.

Table 3. Multivariate analysis of parameters predicting a urination response to tolvaptan therapy.

		Urine Na/K ratio	
		<3.09 (n= 47)	≥3.09 (n = 30)
BUN/Cr ratio	<17.5 (n = 23)	10/12 (83.3%)	8/8 (100.0%)
	≥17.5 (n = 64)	13/33 (39.4%)	19/22 (86.3%)

Notes. BUN/Cr, blood urea nitrogen/creatinine; Na/K, sodium/potassium.

Table 4. Response to tolvaptan according to BUN/Cr and urine Na/K ratios.

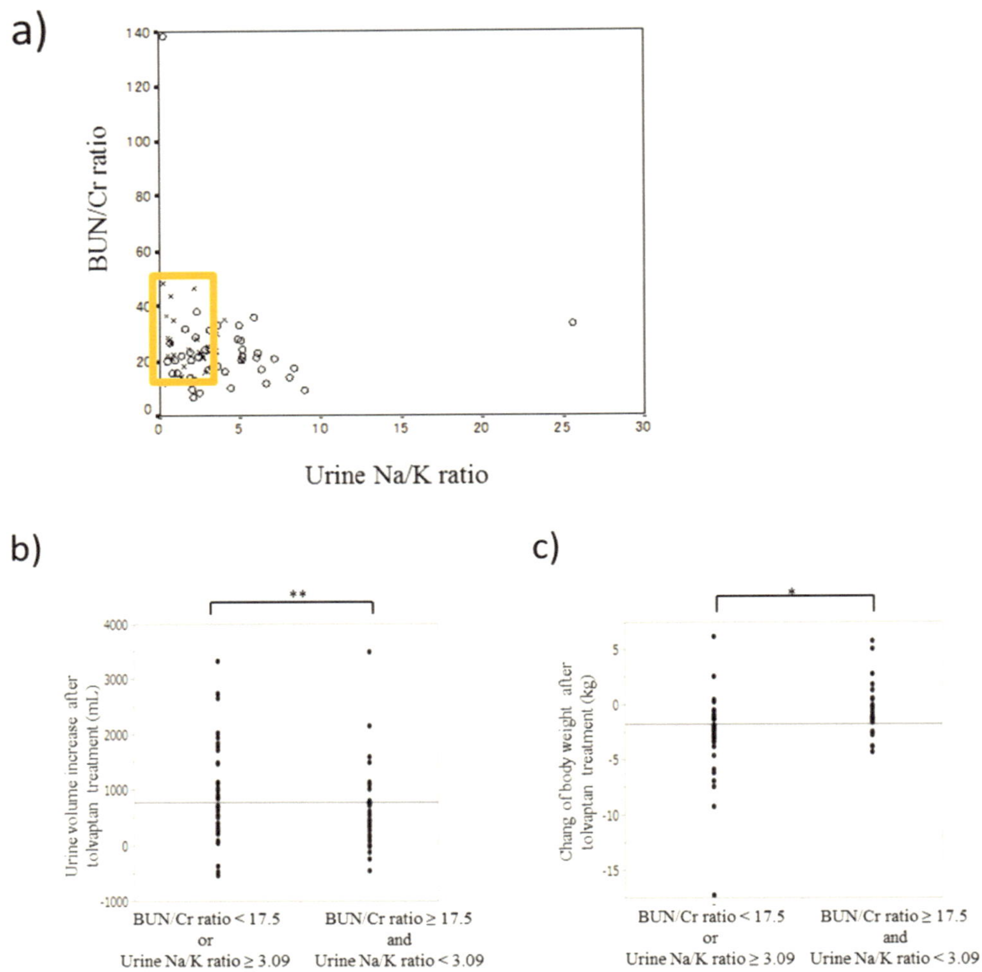

Figure 2. Distributions of the BUN/Cr ratio and urinary Na/K ratio and changes in urine volume and body weight. (a) Distributions of the BUN/Cr ratio and urinary Na/K ratio according to the tolvaptan response. Circle, responder, cross, nonresponder; framed square, BUN/Cr ratio ≥17.5, and urine Na/K ratio <3.09. Changes in (b) urine volume and (c) body weight in patients with and those without a BUN/Cr ratio ≥17.5 and urine Na/K ratio <3.09. Patients without a BUN/Cr ratio ≥17.5 and urine Na/K ratio <3.09 showed greater reductions in urine volume after 1 day (b) and in body weight after 1 week of treatment (c). BUN/Cr, blood urea nitrogen/creatinine; Na/K, sodium/potassium, *p < 0.01, **p < 0.05.

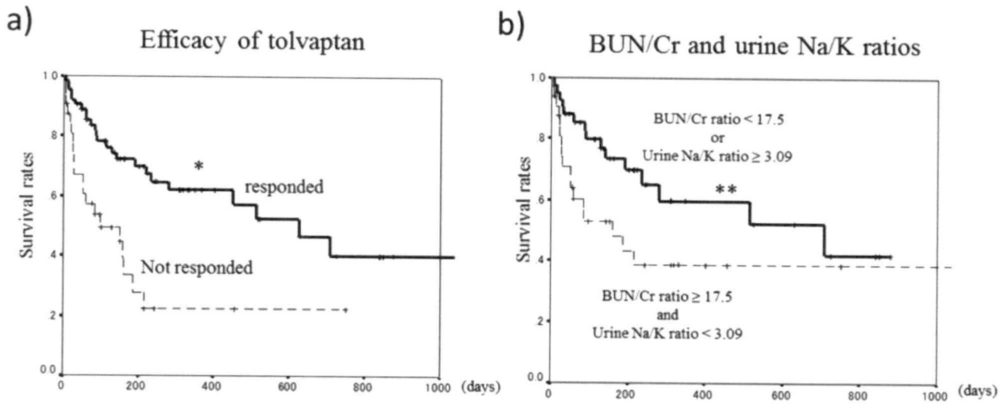

a)

	Total	Number of events	Number censored	Percent censored
———	65	24	41	63.1
- - - -	32	20	12	37.5
Overall	97	44	53	54.6

b)

	Total	Number of events	Number censored	Percent censored
———	42	15	27	64.3
- - - -	33	17	16	48.5
Overall	75	32	43	57.3

Figure 3. Survival rate of patients with and without a response to tolvaptan and the BUN/Cr and urine Na/K ratios. Patients who responded to tolvaptan therapy (a) and who did not have a BUN/Cr ratio ≥17.5 or urine Na/K ratio <3.09 (b) showed a significantly higher survival rate compared with nonresponders. BUN/Cr, blood urea nitrogen/creatinine; Na/K, sodium/potassium, *$p < 0.01$, **$p < 0.05$.

criteria of a BUN/Cr ratio <17.5 and urine Na/K ratio ≥3.09 achieved high tolvaptan response rates ($n = 8$, 100%; **Table 4**). In contrast, patients with a BUN/Cr ratio ≥17.5 and urine Na/K ratio <3.09 exhibited an extremely poor response (**Figure 2a**, framed area). In those patients who did not meet these criteria, urination and body weight reductions were observed (**Figure 2b** and **c**).

3.3. Prognosis after tolvaptan treatment

Regarding the mortality rate, 44 subjects died (45.4%). The survival rate was higher in patients who responded to tolvaptan therapy, as estimated by the Kaplan–Meier analysis (**Figure 3a**, $p < 0.01$). Patients with a BUN/Cr ratio <17.5 or urine Na/K ratio ≥3.09 showed a significantly higher survival rate than that of those who did not meet these criteria (**Figure 3b**, $p < 0.05$).

After 1 week of treatment, 70.1% of the patients achieved a normal serum Na level. These patients showed a significantly higher survival rate ($p < 0.05$). Among the patients with an initial Na level of <135 mEq/L ($n = 38$), 50.0% achieved a normal Na level after tolvaptan therapy and showed a significantly higher survival rate than that of patients without normalized Na levels ($p < 0.05$).

4. Discussion

The results suggest that the initial BUN/Cr and urine Na/K ratios and a normalized serum Na level after 1 week of treatment is predictive of a tolvaptan response in cirrhosis patients. The patients showing a response to tolvaptan in terms of increased urination or serum Na level had prolonged survival and a better prognosis.

Representative factors predicting a response to tolvaptan are shown in **Table 5**. Free water clearance [14], aquaporin-2/AVP [15], and urinary Na excretion [16] were reported to be predictors of a tolvaptan response in patients with cirrhosis. The combination of BUN/Cr and urine Na/K ratios was the first reported predictor of a tolvaptan response.

Regarding prognosis, tolvaptan reduced the rate of inhospital mortality [17] and evidenced longer mortality same as other diuretics in heart failure patients [18], although no study has assessed these parameters in cirrhotic patients. In our study, patients with a BUN/Cr <17.5 or urine Na/K ≥3.09 showed high response rates. Approximately 50.0% of tolvaptan-treated patients reached a normal serum Na level after 1 week of tolvaptan therapy. Patients who responded to tolvaptan exhibited prolonged survival compared with those who did not. Tolvaptan may improve the prognosis.

Tolvaptan has been reported to delay the onset of end-stage renal disease and to be associated with a low rate of renal function deterioration [19, 20]. Therefore, early initiation of tolvaptan is recommended to protect renal function and improve prognosis.

However, our study had limitations because hepatocellular carcinoma (HCC) affects the mortality rate of patients with cirrhosis. Therefore, HCC cases must be excluded from prognostic analyses.

Author	Journal	Year	Predictor	Disease
Imamura et al. [21]	Circ J.	2013	Urine osmolality and percentage decrease in urine osmolarity	Heart failure
Imamura et al. [22]	Circ J.	2014	Urine aquaporin-2 (AQP2)/plasma arginine vasopressin	Heart failure
Okayama et al. [23]	Am J Cardiovasc Drugs	2015	Blood urea nitrogen/ creatinine (BUN/Cr) ratio	Heart failure
Shimizu et al. [24]	Nephrology (Carlton)	2015	Urine urea nitrogen/BUN ratio	Heart failure
Iwatani et al. [25]	Nephron	2015	Urine osmolarity	Chronic kidney disease
Miyaaki et al. [14]	Biomed Rep.	2015	Free water clearance	Liver cirrhosis
Nakanishi et al. [15]	J Gastroenterol.	2016	Urinary AQP2/Cr ratio	Liver cirrhosis
Chishina et al. [26]	Dig Dis.	2016	Serum BUN and serum Cr	Liver cirrhosis
Imamura et al. [27]	Int J Mol Sci.	2016	Urine AQP2	Heart failure
Kogiso et al. [13]	Hepatol Res.	2016	Serum BUN/Cr and urine sodium/potassium ratios	Liver cirrhosis

Table 5. Representative predictors of the response to tolvaptan therapy.

5. Conclusion

In addition to the combination of an initial BUN/Cr ratio <17.5 and urine Na/K ratio ≥3.09, a normalized serum Na level after 1 week of tolvaptan therapy was predictive of a favorable outcome in cirrhotic patients with hyponatremia and ascites treated with tolvaptan.

Author details

Tomomi Kogiso*, Kuniko Yamamoto, Mutsuki Kobayashi, Yuichi Ikarashi, Kazuhisa Kodama, Makiko Taniai, Nobuyuki Torii, Etsuko Hashimoto and Katsutoshi Tokushige

*Address all correspondence to: kogiso.ige@twmu.ac.jp

Department of Internal Medicine, Institute of Gastroenterology, Tokyo Women's, Medical University, Shinjuku-ku, Tokyo, Japan

References

[1] Ginés P, Quintero E, Arroyo V, Terés J, Bruguera M, Rimola A, Caballería J, Rodés J, Rozman C. Compensated cirrhosis: Natural history and prognostic factors. Hepatology. 1987;**7**:122-128

[2] Planas R, Montoliu S, Ballesté B, Rivera M, Miquel M, Masnou H, Galeras JA, Giménez MD, Santos J, Cirera I, Morillas RM, Coll S, Solà R. Natural history of patients hospitalized for management of cirrhotic ascites. Clinical Gastroenterology and Hepatology. 2006;**4**:1385-1394. DOI: 10.1016/j.cgh.2006.08.007

[3] Pérez-Ayuso RM, Arroyo V, Planas R, Gaya J, Bory F, Rimola A, Rivera F, Rodés J. Randomized comparative study of efficacy of furosemide versus spironolactone in nonazotemic cirrhosis with ascites. Relationship between the diuretic response and the activity of the renin-aldosterone system. Gastroenterology. 1983;**84**:961-968

[4] Sherlock S, Senewiratne B, Scott A, Walker JG. Complications of diuretic therapy in hepatic cirrhosis. Lancet. 1966;**1**:1049-1052

[5] Fukui H, Saito H, Ueno Y, Uto H, Obara K, Sakaida I, Shibuya A, Seike M, Nagoshi S, Segawa M, Tsubouchi H, Moriwaki H, Kato A, Hashimoto E, Michitaka K, Murawaki T, Sugano K, Watanabe M, Shimosegawa T. Evidence-based clinical practice guidelines for liver cirrhosis 2015. Journal of Gastroenterology. 2016;**51**:629-650. DOI: 10.1007/s00535-016-1216-y.

[6] Sakaida I, Nakajima K, Okita K, Hori M, Izumi T, Sakurai M, Shibasaki Y, Tachikawa S, Tsubouchi H, Oka H, Kobayashi H. Can serum albumin level affect the pharmacological action of tolvaptan in patients with liver cirrhosis? A post hoc analysis of previous clinical trials in Japan. Journal of Gastroenterology. 2015;**50**:1047-1053. DOI: 10.1007/s00535-015-1052-5.

[7] Schrier RW, Arroyo V, Bernardi M, Epstein M, Henriksen JH, Rodés J. Peripheral arterial vasodilation hypothesis: A proposal for the initiation of renal sodium and water retention in cirrhosis. Hepatology. 1988;**8**:1151-1157

[8] Grace JA, Herath CB, Mak KY, Burrell LM, Angus PW. Update on new aspects of the renin-angiotensin system in liver disease: Clinical implications and new therapeutic options. Clinical Science (London). 2012;**123**:225-239. DOI: 10.1042/CS20120030

[9] Okita K, Sakaida I, Okada M, Kaneko A, Chayama K, Kato M, Sata M, Yoshihara H, Ono N, Murawaki Y. A multicenter, open-label, dose-ranging study to exploratively evaluate the efficacy, safety, and dose-response of tolvaptan in patients with decompensated liver cirrhosis. Journal of Gastroenterology. 2010;**45**:979-987. DOI: 10.1007/s00535-010-0240-6

[10] Sakaida I, Yamashita S, Kobayashi T, Komatsu M, Sakai T, Komorizono Y, Okada M, Okita K; ASCITES 14-Day Administration Study Group. Efficacy and safety of a 14-day administration of tolvaptan in the treatment of patients with ascites in hepatic oedema. The Journal of International Medical Research. 2013;**4**:835-847. DOI: 10.1177/0300060513480089

[11] Kogiso T, Tokushige K, Hashimoto E, Ikarashi Y, Kodama K, Taniai M, Torii N, Shiratori K. Safety and efficacy of long-term tolvaptan therapy for decompensated liver cirrhosis. Hepatology Research. 2016;**46**:E194-E200. DOI: 10.1111/hepr.12547

[12] Ohki T, Sato K, Yamada T, Yamagami M, Ito D, Kawanishi K, Kojima K, Seki M, Toda N, Tagawa K. Efficacy of tolvaptan in patients with refractory ascites in a clinical setting. World Journal of Hepatology. 2015;**7**:1685-1693. DOI: 10.4254/wjh.v7.i12.1685

[13] Kogiso T, Yamamoto K, Kobayashi M, Ikarashi Y, Kodama K, Taniai M, Torii N, Hashimoto E, Tokushige K. Response to tolvaptan and its effect on prognosis in cirrhotic patients with ascites. Hepatology Research. 2016. In press. DOI: 10.1111/hepr.12822.

[14] Miyaaki H, Nakamura Y, Ichikawa T, Taura N, Miuma S, Shibata H, Honda T, Nakao K. Predictive value of the efficacy of tolvaptan in liver cirrhosis patients using free water clearance. Biomedical Reports. 2015;**3**:884-886. DOI: 10.3892/br.2015.521

[15] Nakanishi H, Kurosaki M, Hosokawa T, Takahashi Y, Itakura J, Suzuki S, Yasui Y, Tamaki N, Nakakuki N, Takada H, Higuchi M, Komiyama Y, Yoshida T, Takaura K, Hayashi T, Kuwabara K, Sasaki S, Izumi N. Urinary excretion of the water channel aquaporin 2 correlated with the pharmacological effect of tolvaptan in cirrhotic patients with ascites. Journal of Gastroenterology. 2016;**51**:620-627. DOI: 10.1007/s00535-015-1143-3

[16] Uojima H, Kinbara T, Hidaka H, Sung JH, Ichida M, Tokoro S, Masuda S, Takizawa S, Sasaki A, Koizumi K, Egashira H, Kako M. Close correlation between urinary sodium excretion and response to tolvaptan in liver cirrhosis patients with ascites. Hepatology Research. 2017;**47**:E14-E21. DOI: 10.1111/hepr.12716

[17] Yoshioka K, Matsue Y, Kagiyama N, Yoshida K, Kume T, Okura H, Suzuki M, Matsumura A, Yoshida K, Hashimoto Y. Recovery from hyponatremia in acute phase is associated with better in-hospital mortality rate in acute heart failure syndrome. Journal of Cardiology. 2016;**67**:406-411. DOI: 10.1016/j.jjcc.2015.12.004

[18] Suzuki S, Yoshihisa A, Yamaki T, Sugimoto K, Kunii H, Nakazato K, Abe Y, Saito T, Ohwada T, Suzuki H, Saitoh S, Kubota I, Takeishi Y. Long-term effects and prognosis in acute heart failure treated with tolvaptan: The AVCMA trial. BioMed Research International. 2014;**2014**:704289. DOI: 10.1155/2014/704289

[19] Kimura K, Momose T, Hasegawa T, Morita T, Misawa T, Motoki H, Izawa A, Ikeda U. Early administration of tolvaptan preserves renal function in elderly patients with acute decompensated heart failure. Journal of Cardiology. 2016;**67**:399-405. DOI: 10.1016/j.jjcc.2015.09.020

[20] Mori T, Ohsaki Y, Oba-Yabana I, Ito S. Diuretic usage for protection against end-organ damage in liver cirrhosis and heart failure. Hepatology Research. 2017;**47**:11-22. DOI: 10.1111/hepr.12700

[21] Imamura T, Kinugawa K, Minatsuki S, Muraoka H, Kato N, Inaba T, Maki H, Shiga T, Hatano M, Yao A, Kyo S, Komuro I. Urine osmolality estimated using urine urea nitrogen, sodium and creatinine can effectively predict response to tolvaptan in decompensated heart failure patients. Circulation Journal. 2013;**77**:1208-1213

[22] Imamura T, Kinugawa K, Fujino T, Inaba T, Maki H, Hatano M, Yao A, Komuro I. Increased urine aquaporin-2 relative to plasma arginine vasopressin is a novel marker of response to tolvaptan in patients with decompensated heart failure. Circulation Journal. 2014;**78**:2240-2249

[23] Okayama D, Suzuki T, Shiga T, Minami Y, Tsuruoka S, Hagiwara N. Blood urea nitrogen/creatinine ratio and response to tolvaptan in patients with decompensated heart failure: A retrospective analysis. American Journal of Cardiovascular Drugs. 2015;**15**:289-293. DOI: 10.1007/s40256-015-0121-8

[24] Shimizu K, Doi K, Imamura T, Noiri E, Yahagi N, Nangaku M, Kinugawa K. Ratio of urine and blood urea nitrogen concentration predicts the response of tolvaptan in congestive heart failure. Nephrology (Carlton). 2015;**20**:405-412

[25] Iwatani H, Kawabata H, Sakaguchi Y, Yamamoto R, Hamano T, Rakugi H, Isaka Y. Urine osmolarity predicts the body weight-reduction response to tolvaptan in chronic kidney disease patients: A retrospective, observational study. Nephron. 2015;**130**:8-12. DOI: 10.1159/000381859

[26] Chishina H, Hagiwara S, Nishida N, Ueshima K, Sakurai T, Ida H, Minami Y, Takita M, Kono M, Minami T, Iwanishi M, Umehara Y, Watanabe T, Komeda Y, Arizumi T, Kudo M. Clinical factors predicting the effect of tolvaptan for refractory ascites in patients with decompensated liver cirrhosis. Digestive Diseases and Sciences. 2016;**34**:659-664. DOI: 10.1159/000448828

[27] Imamura T, Kinugawa K. Urine aquaporin-2: A promising marker of response to the arginine vasopressin type-2 antagonist, tolvaptan in patients with congestive heart failure. International Journal of Molecular Sciences. 2016;**17**(105):1-7. DOI: 10.3390/ijms17010105

Chapter 8

Non-pharmacological Treatment of Ascites

Asma Alnajjar, Faisal Abaalkhail, Tala Beidas,
Mohamed R. Abdelfattah and Hussien Elsiesy

Additional information is available at the end of the chapter

http://dx.doi.org/10.5772/intechopen.70511

Abstract

Diuretics are considered the first-line pharmacological treatment option for ascites. Diuretic treatment begins with spironolactone and furosemide. Non-pharmacological options include salt restriction, large-volume paracentesis (LVP), transjugular intrahepatic portosystemic shunt (TIPS), and peritoneovenous shunt. Ascites can be mobilized if renal sodium excretion tops 78 mmol daily (88 mmol–10 mmol daily) after restricting sodium intake to 88 mmol/day (about 2000 mg/day). The majority of patients with cirrhotic ascites respond to a combination of sodium restriction and diuretics such as spironolactone and furosemide (90%). Ascites that does not respond to sodium restriction and high-dose diuretic treatment (400 mg/day of spironolactone and 160 mg/day of furosemide) or following paracentesis is labeled refractory. Refractory ascites can be managed with large-volume paracentesis or transjugular intrahepatic portosystemic shunt. Peritoneovenous shunting is considered as a third-line treatment option after all other measures such as diuretics, large-volume paracentesis, or transjugular intrahepatic portosystemic shunt deemed unsuccessful or contraindicated. It has a high rate of shunt obstruction.

Keywords: ascites, treatment, TIPS, paracentesis, non-pharmacological

1. Introduction

According to the European Association for the Study of the Liver [1], management of ascites is based on grading and the patient's clinical presentation. Grade 1 ascites (mild ascites identified by ultrasound) require no treatment. Grade 2 ascites (moderate ascites with moderate abdominal distention) require sodium restriction and diuretics. Grade 3 ascites (gross ascites with marked abdominal distention) necessitate large-volume paracentesis (LVP) followed by both sodium restriction and diuretics. In addition, treatment depends on the underlying cause. Ascites with high serum-ascites albumin gradient (SAAG) is caused by portal hypertension and is managed with sodium restriction and diuretics [2]. On the contrary, treatment of ascites with low SAAG is achieved by managing the causative pathology [2]. In this chapter, the role for non-pharmacological therapeutic options such as sodium restriction, paracentesis, transjugular intrahepatic portosystemic shunt (TIPS), and peritoneovenous shunt (PVS) in the management of ascites will be discussed (**Table 1**).

	Treatment	Comment
1	Salt restriction	• First-line therapy along with diuretics
2	LVP	• Needs albumin infusion to prevent PICD
3	TIPS	• Encephalopathy is the main complication • High patency rate with PTFE-coated stent • Proper selection prevents hepatic decompensation
4	PVS	• Very limited use in clinical practice • High occlusion rate

Table 1. Non-pharmacological therapy for ascites due to liver cirrhosis.

2. Dietary sodium restriction

In ascites, the decreased sodium excretion leads to a positive sodium balance [3]. Dietary sodium restriction, along with diuretics, is considered the first-line treatment options for patients with cirrhotic ascites [2]. Limiting sodium intake to 88 mmol/day (about 2000 mg/day) is recommended [4]. Cirrhotic patients without fever or diarrhea have about less than 10 mmol of non-renal sodium excretion daily [5]. Ascites can be mobilized if renal sodium excretion tops 78 mmol daily (88 mmol–10 mmol daily) [2]. Adherence to dietary sodium restriction can be assessed by 24-hour urinary sodium, random urinary sodium concentrations, or urine sodium/potassium ratio [2]. A urine sodium/potassium ratio >1 with no evidence of weight loss indicates nonadherence [6]. Unfortunately, only 10–20% of the patients improve with sodium restriction, necessitating the additional use of diuretics for better mobilization of ascites [3]. Moreover, strict limitations of sodium intake may exacerbate the already existing state of malnutrition these patients already have [7].

3. Large-volume paracentesis

Nearly 90% of patients with cirrhotic ascites respond to a combination of sodium restriction and diuretics (spironolactone and furosemide) [8]. About 5–10% become refractory to the abovementioned treatment [9]. Ascites that does not respond to sodium restriction and high-dose diuretic treatment (400 mg/day of spironolactone and 160 mg/day of furosemide) or following paracentesis is labeled refractory [10]. Patients who require more than three admissions annually have recurrent ascites [11]. Moreover, patients with refractory ascites have a low average survival rate of about 6 months [12]. Patients with either refractory ascites or grade 3 ascites require LVP [12]. LVP is a procedure performed in the office-based setting by inserting a needle in the left iliac fossa or by inserting a peritoneal drain for duration of 3 days [12, 13]. Of notice, there is no increased risk of spontaneous bacterial peritonitis (SBP) with the latter method [14]. Quintero et al. concluded that removal of 5 l of ascites by paracentesis in patients with pitting edema caused the fluid to shift from the periphery and redistribute [15]. Moreover, both Gentile et al. [16] and Pinto et al. [17] agreed on the safety of tapping 5 l of ascetic fluid without the hemodynamic changes that follow the procedure, such as a drop in diastolic pressure, aldosterone release, and decreased sodium excretion. With large-volume paracentesis alone, decreased blood volume more than 3 hours after paracentesis is expected to happen as right atrial pressure, Pulmonary capillary wedge pressure (PCWP), and cardiac output markedly drop [18]. Removing a considerable amount of ascetic fluid increases the risk for paracentesis-induced circulatory dysfunction (PICD) [19]. PICD is associated with increased mortality rate at 6 months [20]. Administering 8 g of intravenous albumin/liter of ascetic fluid removed prevents paracentesis-induced circulatory dysfunction (PICD) following drainage of more than 5 l of ascetic fluid [1, 6, 21]. Gines et al. evaluated the role of IV albumin administration in patients who underwent LVP. Only 2% of patients who received IV albumin experienced renal dysfunction and hyponatremia in contrast to those who did not receive IV albumin (21%) [21]. In PICD, vasodilation leads to activation of the renin-angiotensin system in an attempt to restore systemic vascular resistance [22]. Renal dysfunction, vasopressin release and water retention, hypervolemic hyponatremia, and underfilling are consequences [22]. Interestingly, using 4 g (half the dose) of IV albumin in prevention of PICD was as effective as using 8 g [23]. Studies also reported the role of terlipressin, a V1 receptor agonist, as a vasoconstrictor in preventing the neurohumoral responses following paracentesis [24, 25]. Moreau et al. compared the actions of both IV albumin and terlipressin in inhibiting arterial vasodilation, and both were found to be effective [24]. In contrast to albumin, terlipressin is much cheaper [24].

4. Transjugular intrahepatic portosystemic shunt

TIPS could be a substitute for LVP in patients who require more than three LVPs monthly or those with recurrent ascites [12]. In TIPS, a communication is created between the portal and outflow hepatic veins, aiming at lowering portal venous pressure and subsequent activation of renin-angiotensin system [26]. Ascites usually resolves without the need for diuretics or sodium restriction following TIPS insertion, as patients easily excrete sodium; however, diuretics may be needed for few months after TIPS placement [27–29]. Moreover, norepinephrine, plasma renin, and aldosterone activities decrease following TIPS insertion, leading to improved renal function in patients with cirrhosis [27–29]. The main indication for TIPS in cirrhotic patients is acute variceal bleeding not responding to endoscopic and medical therapy, refractory ascites, or for secondary prevention of gastric variceal bleeding [2]. Several studies compared the role of TIPS to LVP with IV albumin infusion. Unfortunately, the results of the studies showed that patients with TIPS insertion had a worse prognosis in patients with refractory ascites [30–33]. This may be explained by poor patient selection for TIPS. However, patients who have TIPS insertion with polytetrafluoroethylene (PTFE)-covered stents had better outcomes and stent patency compared to those with bare-metal stents [34, 35]. Model for end-stage liver disease (MELD) is a scoring system for evaluating the severity of chronic liver disease. It was developed initially to predict the 3 months of mortality in patients who had undergone a TIPS procedure [36] and was subsequently adopted for prioritizing receipts on the waiting list for liver transplantation [37, 38].

High MELD score [39] and bilirubin levels >3 mg/dl [40, 41] increase mortality rates in patients who had TIPS placement; therefore, good selection of candidates for TIPS is very important for good outcome. Hepatic encephalopathy is the main complication encountered in 25–30% of patients who undergo TIPS, especially older patients [41, 42]. TIPS is contraindicated in patients with severe pulmonary hypertension, portal thrombosis, heart failure, and advanced liver disease (Child-Pugh class C) [3].

5. Peritoneovenous shunts

PVS can be used in the treatment of refractory ascites that needed multiple LVPs or patients who cannot have TIPS placement or liver transplantation [13, 43]. In PVS, a one-way valve tube is created to allow movement of ascites from the positively pressured peritoneum to the superior vena cava through the internal jugular vein in the negatively pressured chest cavity [44]. If central venous pressure gets elevated, the flow is hindered [3]. Most common complication encountered with PVS is obstruction of the shunt [45]. Coagulation disorders, severe cardiac or kidney failure, and loculated ascites are contraindications for PVS [13]. Moreover, PVS is not frequently used due to lack of survival benefit and low shunt patency rate [46, 47]. In addition, sepsis and SBP prompt shunt removal [43]. The abovementioned leaves PVS with very limited use in clinical practice as a treatment option after all other measures such as diuretics, LVP, and TIPS deemed unsuccessful or contraindicated [43, 48, 49].

Author details

Asma Alnajjar[1], Faisal Abaalkhail[1,2], Tala Beidas[1], Mohamed R. Abdelfattah[3] and Hussien Elsiesy[1,2*]

*Address all correspondence to: helsiesy@gmail.com

1 Department of Medicine, Alfaisal University, Riyadh, Saudi Arabia

2 Department of Liver Transplantation, King Faisal Specialist Hospital & Research Center, Riyadh, Saudi Arabia

3 Department of Surgery, University of Alexandria, Faculty of Medicine, Alexandria, Egypt

References

[1] European Association for the Study of the Liver (EASL). Clinical practice guidelines on the management of ascites, spontaneous bacterial peritonitis, and hepatorenal syndrome in cirrhosis. Journal of Hepatology. 2010;**53**(3):397-417

[2] Amer MO, Elsiesy H. In: Tsoulfas G, (editor). Ascites: Causes, Diagnosis, and Treatment, Liver Cirrhosis – Update and Current Challenges. InTech, DOI: 10.5772/intechopen.68868. Available from: https://www.intechopen.com/books/liver-cirrhosis-update-and-current-challenges/ascites-causes-diagnosis-and-treatment

[3] Lenz K, Buder R, Kapun L, Voglmayr M. Treatment and management of ascites and hepatorenal syndrome: An update. Therapeutic Advances in Gastroenterology. 2015;**8**(2):83-100

[4] Runyon BA. Care of patients with ascites. New England Journal of Medicine. 1994;**330**(5):337-342

[5] Eisenmenger WJ, et al. Electrolyte studies on patients with cirrhosis of the liver. Journal of Clinical Investigation. 1950;**29**(11):1491-1499

[6] Runyon BA. Management of adult patients with ascites due to cirrhosis: An update. Hepatology. 2009;**49**:2087-2107

[7] Soulsby C, Madden A, Morgan M. The effect of dietary sodium restriction on energy and protein intake. Hepatology. 1997;**26**(Suppl. 382A):1013

[8] Biecker E. Diagnosis and therapy of ascites in liver cirrhosis. World Journal of Gastroenterology: WJG. 2011;**17**(10):1237-1248. DOI: 10.3748/wjg.v17.i10.1237

[9] Moore KP, Aithal GP. Guidelines on the management of ascites in cirrhosis. Gut. 2006;**55**(Suppl. 6):vi1-vi12

[10] Gines P, Angeli P, Lenz K, Moller S, Moore K, Moreau R. EASL clinical practice guidelines on the management of ascites, spontaneous bacterial peritonitis, and hepatorenal syndrome in cirrhosis. Journal of Hepatology. 2010;**53**:397-417

[11] Arroyo V. A new method for therapeutic paracentesis: The automated low flow pump system. Comments in the context of the history of paracentesis. Journal of Hepatology. 2013;**58**:850-852

[12] Pedersen JS, Bendtsen F, Møller S. Management of cirrhotic ascites. Therapeutic Advances in Chronic Disease. 2015;**6**(3):124-137

[13] Moore CM, Van Thiel DH. Cirrhotic ascites review: Pathophysiology, diagnosis and management. World Journal of Hepatology. 2013;**5**(5):251-263

[14] Van Thiel DH, Moore CM, Garcia M, George M, Nadir A. Continuous peritoneal drainage of large-volume ascites. Digestive Diseases and Sciences. 2011;**56**:2723-2727

[15] Quintero E, Ginés P, Arroyo V, Rimola A, Bory F, Planas R, Viver J, Cabrera J, Rodés J. Paracentesis versus diuretics in the treatment of cirrhotics with tense ascites. Lancet. 1985;**1**:611-612

[16] Gentile S, Angelico M, Bologna E, Capocaccia L. Clinical, biochemical, and hormonal changes after a single, large-volume paracentesis in cirrhosis with ascites. The American Journal of Gastroenterology. 1989;**84**:279-284

[17] Pinto PC, Amerian J, Reynolds TB. Large-volume paracentesis in nonedematous patients with tense ascites: Its effect on intravascular volume. Hepatology. 1988;**8**:207-210

[18] Panos MZ, Moore K, Vlavianos P, Chambers JB, Anderson JV, Gimson AE, Slater JD, Rees LH, Westaby D, Williams R. Single, total paracentesis for tense ascites: Sequential hemodynamic changes and right atrial size. Hepatology. 1990;**11**:662-667

[19] Ginès P, Arroyo V. Paracentesis in the management of cirrhotic ascites. Journal of Hepatology. 1993;**17**(Suppl. 2):S14-S18

[20] Planas R, Ginès P, Arroyo V, Llach J, Panés J, Vargas V, Salmerón JM, Ginès A, Toledo C, Rimola A. Dextran-70 versus albumin as plasma expanders in cirrhotic patients with tense ascites treated with total paracentesis. Results of a randomized study. Gastroenterology. 1990;**99**:1736-1744

[21] Gines P, Tito L, Arroyo V, Planas R, Panes J, Viver J, et al. Randomized comparative study of therapeutic paracentesis with and without intravenous albumin in cirrhosis. Gastroenterology. 1988;**94**:1493-1502

[22] Ruiz-del-Arbol L, Monescillo A, Jimenéz W, Garcia-Plaza A, Arroyo V, Rodés J. Paracentesis-induced circulatory dysfunction: Mechanism and effect on hepatic hemodynamics in cirrhosis. Gastroenterology. 1997;**113**:579-586

[23] Alessandria C, Elia C, Mezzabotta L, Risso A, Andrealli A, Spandre M, Morgando A, Marzano A, Rizzetto M. Prevention of paracentesis-induced circulatory dysfunction in cirrhosis: Standard vs half albumin doses. A prospective, randomized, unblinded pilot study. Digestive and Liver Disease. 2011;**43**:881-886

[24] Moreau R, Asselah T, Condat B, de Kerguenec C, Pessione F, Bernard B, Poynard T, Binn M, Grangé JD, Valla D, Lebrec D. Comparison of the effect of terlipressin and albumin on arterial blood volume in patients with cirrhosis and tense ascites treated by paracentesis: A randomised pilot study. Gut. 2002;**50**:90-94

[25] Fimiani B, Guardia DD, Puoti C, D'Adamo G, Cioffi O, Pagano A, Tagliamonte MR, Izzi A. The use of terlipressin in cirrhotic patients with refractory ascites and normal renal function: A multicentric study. European Journal of Internal Medicine. 2011;**22**:587-590

[26] Rossle M, Siegerstetter V, Huber M, Ochs A. The first decade of the transjugular intrahepatic portosystemic shunt (TIPS): State of the art. Liver. 1998;**18**:73-89

[27] Wong F, et al. The mechanism of the initial natriuresis after transjugular intrahepatic portosystemic shunt. Gastroenterology. 1997;**112**(3):899-907

[28] Guevara M, et al. Transjugular intrahepatic portosystemic shunt in hepatorenal syndrome: Effects on renal function and vasoactive systems. Hepatology. 1998;**28**(2):416-422

[29] Gerbes AL, et al. Renal effects of transjugular intrahepatic portosystemic shunt in cirrhosis: Comparison of patients with ascites, with refractory ascites, or without ascites. Hepatology. 1998;**28**(3):683-688

[30] Gines P, Uriz J, Calahorra B, García-Tsao G, Kamath P, Ruiz-del-Arbol L, et al. Transjugular intrahepatic portosystemic shunting versus paracentesis plus albumin for refractory ascites in cirrhosis. Gastroenterology. 2002;**123**:1839-1847

[31] Lebrec D, Giuily N, Hadengue A, Vilgrain V, Moreau R, Poynard T, et al. Transjugular intrahepatic portosystemic shunts: Comparison with paracentesis in patients with cirrhosis and refractory ascites: A randomized trial. Journal of Hepatology. 1996;**25**:135-144

[32] Rössle M, Ochs A, Gulberg V, Siegerstetter V, Holl J, Deibert P, et al. A comparison of paracentesis and transjugular intrahepatic portosystemic shunting in patients with ascites. The New England Journal of Medicine. 2000;**342**:1701-1707

[33] Sanyal A, Genning C, Reddy K, Wong F, Kowdley K, Benner K, et al. The North America study for the treatment of refractory ascites. Gastroenterology. 2003;**124**:634-641

[34] Bureau C, et al. Improved clinical outcome using polytetrafluoroethylene-coated stents for TIPS: Results of a randomized study. Gastroenterology. 2004;**126**(2):469-475

[35] Angermayr B, et al. Survival in patients undergoing transjugular intrahepatic portosystemic shunt: ePTFE-covered stentgrafts versus bare stents. Hepatology. 2003;**38**(4):1043-1050

[36] Malinchoc M, Kamath PS, Gordon FD, Peine CJ, Rank J, ter Borg PC. A model to predict poor survival in patients undergoing transjugular intrahepatic portosystemic shunts. Hepatology. 2000 Apr;**31**(4):864-871

[37] Kamath PS, Wiesner RH, Malinchoc M, et al. A model to predict survival in patients with end-stage liver disease. Hepatology. 2001 Feb;**33**(2):464-470

[38] Kamath PS, Kim WR, Advanced Liver Disease Study Group. The model for end-stage liver disease (MELD). Hepatology. 2007 Mar;**45**(3):797-805

[39] Angemayr B, Cejna M, Karnel F, Gschwantler M, Koenig F, Pidlich J, et al. Child-pugh versus MELD score in predicting survival in patients undergoing transjugular intrahepatic portosystemic shunt. Gut. 2003;**52**:879-885

[40] Gerbes A, Gülberg V. Benefit of TIPS for patients with refractory ascites or recidivant ascites: Serum bilirubin may make the difference. Hepatology. 2005;**41**:217

[41] Casado M, Bosch J, Garcia-Pagan J, Bru C, Banares R, Bandi J, et al. Clinical events after transjugular intrahepatic portosystemic shunt: Correlation with hemodynamic findings. Gastroenterology. 1998;**114**:1296-1303

[42] Sanyal A, Freedman A, Shiffman M, Purdum P, 3rd, Luketic V, Cheatham A. Portosystemic encephalopathy after transjugular intrahepatic portosystemic shunt: Results of a prospective controlled study. Hepatology. 1994;**20**:46-55

[43] Moskovitz M. The peritoneovenous shunt: Expectations and reality. The American Journal of Gastroenterology. 1990;**85**:917-929

[44] LeVeen H, Christoudias G, Ip M, Luft R, Flak G, Grosberg S. Peritoneo-venous shunting for ascites. Annals of Surgery. 1974;**180**:580-591

[45] Rodes J. Pathogenesis and treatment of ascites. Journal of Internal Medicine. 1996;**240**(3): 111-114

[46] Stanley MM, et al. Peritoneovenous shunting as compared with medical treatment in patients with alcoholic cirrhosis and massive ascites. Veterans Administration Cooperative Study on treatment of alcoholic cirrhosis with ascites. New England Journal of Medicine. 1989;**321**(24):1632-1638

[47] Gines P, et al. Paracentesis with intravenous infusion of albumin as compared with peritoneovenous shunting in cirrhosis with refractory ascites. The New England Journal of Medicine. 1991;**325**(12):829-835

[48] Boyer TD, Haskal ZJ. The role of transjugular intrahepatic portosystemic shunt (TIPS) in the management of portal hypertension: Update 2009. Hepatology. 2010;**51**:306

[49] Runyon BA. Ascites and spontaneous bacterial peritonitis. In: Feldman M, Friedman LS, Brandt LJ, editors. Sleisenger and Fordtran's Gastrointestinal and Liver Disease. 9th ed. Philadelphia, PA: Saunders; 2010

Chapter 9

Ascites in Ovarian Cancer Progression: Opportunities for Biomarker Discovery and New Avenues for Targeted Therapies

Isabelle Matte, Paul Bessette and Alain Piché

Additional information is available at the end of the chapter

http://dx.doi.org/10.5772/intechopen.70993

Abstract

Until recently, ovarian cancer research has mainly focused on the tumor cell themselves ignoring for the most part the surrounding tumor environment. However, one of the major conceptual advances in oncology over the last few years has been the appreciation that major aspects of cancer biology are influenced by the tumor environment. Malignant ascites accumulates in the peritoneal cavity during ovarian cancer progression and constitutes a unique pro-inflammatory tumor environment providing a framework that orchestrates cellular and molecular changes contributing to aggressiveness and disease progression. The composition of ascites, which includes cellular and acellular components, constantly adapts during the course of the disease in response to various cellular cues originating from both tumor and stromal cells. Increasing evidence now supports an active role of ascites in the progression of ovarian cancer. Although much work is still needed to fully understand the contribution of ascites to ovarian cancer aggressiveness, this tumor environment potentially provides a wealth of opportunities for translational research including biomarker discovery and novel therapeutic target identification. In this review, we discuss recent advances in our understanding of ascites pathophysiology, the characterization of its cellular and acellular contents, the intercellular crosstalks, and how these data can be used to improve the outcome of ovarian cancer.

Keywords: ascites, cytokines, ovarian cancer, progression, metastasis

1. Introduction

Epithelial ovarian cancer (EOC) is the fifth leading cause of cancer-related death among women in the Western world [1]. Early stage diseases are difficult to detect because of the location and size of ovaries and fallopian tubes, the lack of specific symptoms and the absence of reliable screening methods. Consequently, most women with EOC display advanced diseases (stage III/IV) with metastases throughout the pelvic and peritoneal cavities, as well as large amount of ascites, when they seek medical care [2, 3]. The presence of large volume of ascites correlates with poor prognosis and pelvic and peritoneal metastases [4, 5]. EOC encompasses five histopathological subtypes with unique characteristics: high-grade serous carcinoma (HGSC), low-grade serous carcinoma (LGSC), endometrioid carcinoma (EC), mucinous carcinoma (MC), and clear cell carcinoma [6, 7]. High-grade serous ovarian carcinoma (HGSOC) is by far the most common subtype and development of malignant ascites during the course of the disease is particularly common with this subtype [3]. Due to the accumulation of large volume, ascites can be debilitating for patients causing pain, early satiety and respiratory distress [8]. The standard of care for women with high-grade serous ovarian carcinoma (HGSOC) consists of debulking surgery together with platinum-based combination chemotherapy resulting in a median progression-free survival (PFS) of 16–22 months and a 5-year survival rate of 10–30% [1, 9]. This high mortality rate results from the biologic complexity of EOC, from the difficulty of resecting multiple peritoneal tumor implants and from the frequent occurrence of drug resistance, whether intrinsic (primary) or acquired (secondary), the latest being the most frequently observed. Treatment options for women with resistant diseases remain very limited and relapsing diseases are almost always incurable. In contrast, women with localized disease (tumor limited to the primary site) have a 95% 5-year survival [3]. Therefore, it is essential to gain a better understanding of the mechanisms involved in EOC dissemination and how the tumor environment participates to this process in order to develop novel therapeutic approaches that target crucial steps involved in cancer dissemination that could improve long-term survival.

In most human cancers, the tumor microenvironment is heavily altered compared to its normal counterpart [10, 11]. The importance of the tumor microenvironment in cancer progression is now well appreciated. Indeed, bidirectional communications between tumor cells and their surrounding environment influence disease initiation and progression and patient prognosis [12]. In response to evolving environmental conditions and signals from tumor and stromal cells, the surrounding tumor environment is continually changing over the course of cancer progression, underscoring the need to understand how the environment drives the metastatic process. As opposed to the surrounding microenvironment in solid tumors, malignant ascites constitutes a unique form of environment. Recent evidence suggest that ascites plays a major role in tumor progression, emphasizing the necessity to understand its pathophysiology and its impact on the biology of tumor cells, including its role in drug resistance, spheroid formation, tumor dissemination and progression. Here, we discuss the recent advances in our understanding of the role of ascites in ovarian cancer progression. In particular, we address its effects on spheroid formation, dissemination, chemoresistance and metastasis. Pinpointing key molecules in ascites that promote EOC dissemination and progression will provide new strategies to improve EOC survival.

2. What is the tumor environment of ascites

As previously mentioned, EOC progression is characterized by the progressive accumulation of peritoneal fluids, which presumably provides a supportive local environment. Because of its large volume (up to 10 L), its high cell density and lack of anchorage support for cells, the accumulation of peritoneal effusions occurring during EOC progression can be seen as a particular environment. The pathophysiology of ascites accumulation involves decreased clearance of peritoneal fluids, blockade of lymphatic channels drainage, increased permeability of capillaries due in large part to vascular endothelial growth factor (VEGF) [13, 14], decreased protein levels in blood, and decreased hepatic clearance. Ascites is characterized by cellular and acellular fractions. The cellular fraction is populated by a heterogeneous mixture of tumor and stromal cells, which includes mesothelial-derived cells, adipocytes, endothelial and immune cells. These stromal cells account for >99% of the cellular composition of ascites which contrast with the stromal content of tumor tissue which has a median relative proportion of 50% [15]. In solid tumors, stromal cells significantly contribute to malignant progression. In particular, cancer-associated fibroblasts (CAFs) promote cell survival, growth and progression by expressing a pro-inflammatory gene signature leading to secretion of a number of growth factors, including transforming growth factor-β1 (TGF β1), IL-6, CSCL1, and CXCL2 among others [16]. By analogy, stromal cells found in malignant ascites could play a similar role in ovarian cancer progression. Indeed, recent studies suggest that stromal cells in ascites facilitate tumor growth, survival and invasion [17–19].

The acellular fraction of ascites constitutes a dynamic reservoir of cytokines, growth factors, bioactive lipids and extracellular matrix (ECM) components that may have either pro- or anti-tumorigenic effects [20–25]. A number of factors in ascites, including CCL18, HGF, LPA and VEGF, have been shown to promote cell migration, invasion and tumorigenesis [20, 26–29].

3. Cellular contents: contribution to EOC metastasis

The origin and phenotype of the stromal cells in ascites is still not well understood. However, ascites is characteristically populated by mesothelial cells [30]. Mesothelial cells exfoliate from the peritoneal lining and accumulate in ascites [31]. Upon sustained inflammation, mesothelial cells lose their epithelial-like characteristics, including dissolution of cell-cell junctions and their apical-basolateral polarity, and acquired a mesenchymal phenotype (mesothelial-to-mesenchymal transition (MMT) giving rise to myofibroblastic-like cells, which are characterized by increased migration and invasion capacities [32]. Lineage-tracing experiments suggest that a sizeable subpopulation of cancer-associated fibroblasts (CAFs) found in ascites probably originates from mesothelial cells through MMT [33]. Mesothelial-derived CAFs share characteristics with myofibroblasts, such as the expression of alpha-smooth muscle actin (αSMA), fibroblast activation protein-α (FAPα) and fibroblast-specific protein 1 (FSP1) [33]. TGF-β has been implicated in mesothelial cell activation leading to MMT [34]. In EOC ascites, myofibroblastic-like cells are present in aberrantly high numbers and are different from normal mesothelial cells. Once these cells accumulate in ascites they can be "educated" by growth factors and cytokines in the surrounding environment to support tumor growth [19]. Upon stimulation by ascites, myofibroblastic-like cells have been shown to produce dipeptidyl peptidase IV [35], which is a multifunctional protein that have been associate with tumor growth in some context [36]. Exposure of myofibroblastic-like cells to ascites increased the secretion of VEGF and other pro-survival soluble factors [19, 37]. Furthermore, data from our laboratory suggest that ascites stimulates the expression and release of MUC16 from the mesothelial cell membranes [38]. MUC16 is an oncogenic high molecular weight mucin that promotes EOC progression [39–42] and regulates the formation of multicellular spheroids [43]. Therefore, through ascites exposure, myofibroblastic-like cells become a major source of secreted factors, which in turn, further contribute to the evolution of the tumor environment. This dynamic interaction between the surrounding environment and stromal cells provides favorable conditions for tumor progression.

In addition to the complex nature of stromal cells present in ascites, this environment also appears to contain distinct populations of tumor cells displaying different phenotypic characteristics. A population of non-adherent tumor cells in 2D cultures expressing E-cadherin, EpCAM, CA125, Oct4 and STAT3 were particularly associated with diseases recurrence [44]. Tumor cells are shed from the primary tumor and aggregate in ascites. Exfoliated tumor cells will form free-floating multicellular spheroids in ascites, which range from 50 to 750 μM in size [45]. These multicellular spheroids probably represent the invasive and metastasis-forming intermediate [46]. In addition, aggregation of tumor cells is essential for anchorage-independent growth and survival. Indeed, once suspended in the peritoneal fluid, cancer cells must resist anoikis, a specialized form of apoptosis triggered by a lack of attachment to other cells or to the extracellular matrix (EMC). Recently, we have characterized multicellular spheroids from HGSOC ascites. Interestingly, we found that these spheroids contained one

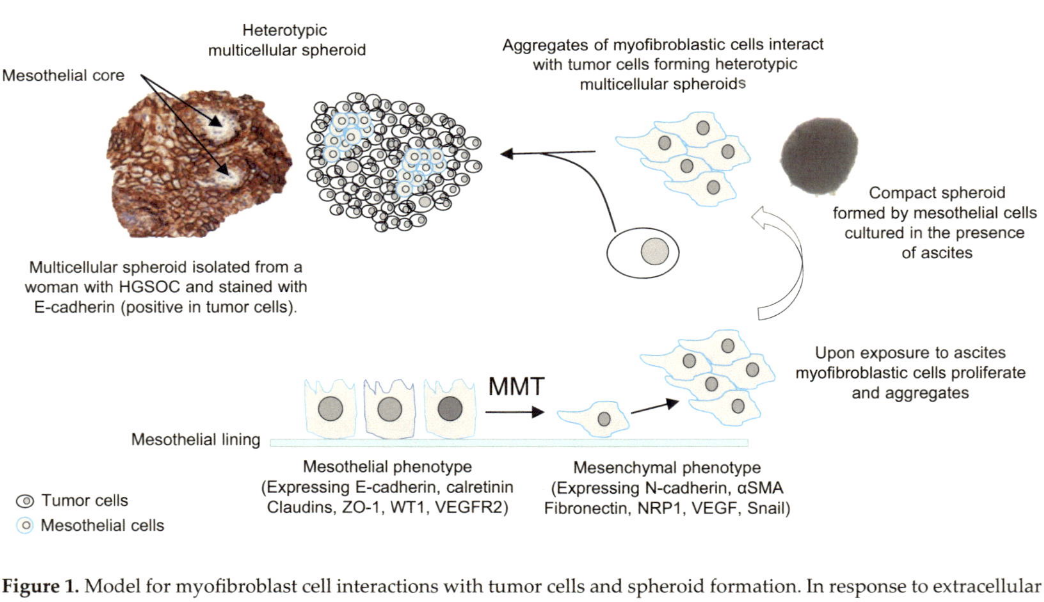

Figure 1. Model for myofibroblast cell interactions with tumor cells and spheroid formation. In response to extracellular cues in the local environment, particularly TGF-β1, mesothelial cells lining the peritoneum undergo a mesothelial-to-mesenchymal transition (MMT) characterized by dissolution of cell-cell junctions, actin reorganization and stress fiber formation. This mesenchymal phenotype is characterized by increased migration and invasion. MMT enables cells to exfoliate from the peritoneum into the existing peritoneal fluid. Unpublished results from our laboratory suggest that, upon exposure to malignant ascites, myofibroblastic-like cells aggregate to form very compact spheroids. These myofibroblastic-like cell aggregates interact with exfoliated tumor cells to form heterotypic multicellular spheroids. Mesothelial cells located in the center of spheroids may provide initial matrix support for EOC cells to avoid anoikis. Extracellular cues from the surrounding environment can induce the secretion of prosurvival factors in mesothelial cells.

or more cores of myofibroblastic-like cells encased in a shell of tumor cells suggesting that free-floating tumor and stromal cells in peritoneal effusions can interact with each other to form heterotypic spheroids (**Figure 1**). The analysis of multicellular spheroid cell components isolated from EOC ascites revealed that myofibroblastic-like cells were present in all spheroids studied [47]. Based on data derived from a 3D *in vitro* model, the interaction between myofibroblastic-like cells and tumor cells is mediated, at least in part, by β1-integrin [45, 47]. In addition, β-catenin-regulated ALDH1A1, a known cancer stem cell marker, has also been implicated in the formation of multicellular spheroids [48]. Recent studies suggest that tumor cells possess varying capacity for spheroid formation [45, 47, 49]. A positive correlation has been reported between compact spheroid formation and a mesenchymal phenotype of tumor cells [47, 49]. Therefore, aggressive cancer cell populations (mesenchymal phenotype) could gain a survival advantage through their propensity to form more compact spheroids. Recent data suggest that the presence of myofibroblasts in multicellular spheroids promotes the invasion of tumor cells [50]. These data suggest that spheroid-associated myofibroblasts may play an important role in EOC progression. In addition, these stromal cells may play a role in the early steps of spheroid formation before peritoneal implantation. Myofibroblasts located within the center of spheroids may provide initial matrix support for tumor cells to avoid anoikis. Spheroid-associated myofibroblasts may also secrete factors within the microenvironment of the spheroids that induce signaling events in tumor cells to further inhibit anoikis. Recent data suggest that tumor-associated macrophages (TAMs) may promote spheroid formation and tumor growth in a mouse model [51]. This group found that nearly 80% of macrophages infiltrated in the peritoneal cavity were detected in spheroids. Spheroid-associated TAMs were shown to secrete large amounts of epidermal growth factor (EGF), which leads to upregulation of integrin and ICAM-1 expression in tumor cells to form a positive autocrine feedback loop [51].

4. Cell-free ascites: biomarkers and EOC progression

As mentioned above, the presence of ascites is correlated with poor prognosis. In a study limited to patients with stage III/IV EOC, women without ascites had a 5-year survival rate of 45% compared to 5% for those with ascites [52]. The composition of cell-free ascites is also a major predictor of clinical prognosis. For example, EOC patients with ascites containing high IL-6 levels (>2662 pg/ml) at diagnostic had a worse outcome [53]. In that study, IL-6 was found to be an independent factor for progression-free survival. Patients with EOC and higher IFN-γ expression levels in ascites have shorter disease-free progression and overall survival [54]. Measuring cytokines in ascites may also provide a novel approach to discriminate patients with intrinsic resistance to first-line therapy [55]. The authors found that the combination of serum CA125 and ascites leptin levels was a strong predictor of clinical resistance to first-line therapy. The biochemical composition of ascites, particularly the levels of chemokines, chemokines receptors and growth factors, including CCL2, CXCL1, CXCL5, CXCL8, CXCL12, HGF, TGF-β1 and VEGF, in undifferentiated tumors could explain, to some extent, the aggressive behavior of this histotype [56]. Ascites is therefore an attractive biofluid for biomarker discovery as it is easy and minimally invasive to obtain. There is indeed growing evidence showing that proximal fluids such as ascites are valuable sources for biomarker discovery as they reflect events in ovarian tumorigenesis earlier than in peripheral blood circulation [57, 58]. The concentration of soluble factors is usually much higher in ascites compared to serum, which increases the likelihood of detecting low abundance proteins [24, 57]. In that context, proteomic/peptidomic profiling of ascites has been employed for biomarker discovery [59–61]. Different experimental approaches were used leading to the identification of various sets of biomarkers all of which requiring further validation to determine their true potential. Nonetheless, ascites profiling represents a potentially new approach for much needed new biomarkers in the context of EOC.

Beyond the contribution of specific cell types in ascites, extracellular cues from cell-free ascites have the potential capacity to drive disease progression. Cytokine profiling of EOC ascites has demonstrated elevated levels of various pro-tumorigenic cytokines including adiponectin, CXCL1, CXCL10, CCL2, CCL4, ICAM-1, IL-6, IL-8, IL-10, IL-15, PDGF-BB, RANTES and VEGF [24, 25]. Theses cytokines contribute to create an inflammatory environment that sustains chronic inflammation. Chronic inflammation, in turns, promotes tumor growth and peritoneal spread [62]. IL-6 is probably the best studied cytokine in that context. IL-6 signaling is known to be associated with specific immune and metabolic alterations that lead to cancer cachexia, which is often seen with advanced diseases. IL-6 plays an important role in the development of ascites as well as the spread of EOC through, at least in part, its induction of tumor angiogenesis [63]. In support for the role of IL-6, we found that IL-6 and sIL-6R are significantly higher in ascites obtained from women with advanced diseases compared to women with stage I/II EOC (**Table 1**). VEGF is a well-established factor that increases vascular permeability. VEGF binding to its receptor activates focal adhesion kinase (FAK) which localizes to the cytoplasmic tail of VE-cadherin at endothelial cell-cell junctions. FAK phosphorylates β-catenin, which destabilizes the cell-cell junctions, resulting in increased vascular permeability [64]. Metabolome profiling of ascites has revealed significant differences in fatty acids, cholesterol, ceramide, glycerol-3-phosphate, glucose and glucose-3-phosphate compared to non-cancerous peritoneal effusions [65]. Whether these changes directly contribute to oncogenic signaling or they merely reflect upregulation of pathways of the fatty acid synthesis associated with increased metabolic activity in tumor cells remains to be determined.

There is extensive cellular crosstalks and signaling events between the surrounding environment and tumor cells during EOC dissemination and progression. As a result, ascites is constantly adapting in response to the different cues. In order to characterize the changes in ascites during EOC progression, we have performed cytokine profiling of stage I/II and III/IV serous ascites. As shown in **Table 1**, 29 cytokines/chemokines/growth factors out of 120 tested were present at significantly higher levels in stage III/IV ascites supporting the idea that ascites evolve during EOC progression. Consistent with the critical role of IL-6 in EOC progression, we found several components of the IL-6 trans-signaling system, including IL-6, IL-6 receptor (IL-6R), and soluble glycoprotein 130 (sgp130), elevated in ascites of women with advanced diseases. Factors such as CCL2 have been implicated in CAFs activation [12]. As mentioned above, once stimulated myofibroblastic-like cells in ascites provide a source of secreted factors that support tumorigenesis.

http://dx.doi.org/10.5772/intechopen.70993

Cytokines	Serous Stage I–II RFU[a] (SEM) (n = 2)	Serous Stage III–IV RFU (SEM) (n = 5)	Fold change	*p*
IL-6	1352 (302)	14183 (10619)	10.5	<0.0001
Angiopoietin-2	6293 (4081)	14683 (11235)	9.8	0.0076
IL-10	457 (45)	4220 (3752)	9.2	0.0003
Leptin	561 (102)	4991 (5849)	8.9	0.0031
sTNF RI	828 (260)	5238 (2768)	6.3	<0.0001
uPAR	1092 (488)	6417 (3387)	5.9	<0.0001
CXCL1	2569 (1386)	14926 (12569)	5.8	0.0003
HGF	1017 (212)	5504 (4708)	5.4	0.0004
OPG	978 (394)	3493 (1606)	3.6	<0.0001
CCL2	1918 (480)	8032 (5439)	4.2	0.0001
Fit-3 ligand	739 (129)	3092 (2119)	4.2	0.0001
CCL16	593 (146)	2313 (1713)	3.9	0.0003
CCL7	630 (119)	2366 (2184)	3.8	0.0021
IL-1 R4/ST2	709 (188)	2194 (2078)	3.1	0.0049
CCL22	776 (131)	2301 (1246)	3.0	<0.0001
ICAM-1	4107 (861)	11832 (4961)	2.9	<0.0001
EGFR	871 (239)	2514 (1937)	2.9	0.0013
IGFBP-6	1274 (594)	3668 (1537)	2.9	<0.0001
IL-16	654 (106)	1814 (1738)	2.8	0.0077
CXCL13	679 (98)	1851 (1477)	2.7	0.0022
Axl	1039 (412)	2578 (856)	2.5	<0.0001
CXCL9	773 (103)	1903 (1308)	2.1	0.0017
sTNF RII	2393 (759)	5301 (1694)	2.5	0.0011
Fas	1487 (557)	3779 (3301)	2.5	0.0067
IL-3	734 (191)	1720 (1058)	2.4	0.0006
CCL4	1312 (369)	2739 (1704)	2.2	<0.0001
CCL19	797 (184)	1712 (1521)	2.2	0.0155
IGFBP-1	2827 (1092)	6007 (4692)	2.1	0.0091
IL-6 R	3602 (1009)	7160 (4835)	2.0	0.0048
MIF	2920 (916)	5460 (3396)	1.9	0.0051
sgp130	1510 (359)	2510 (852)	1.7	0.0002
TIMP-1	1189 (233)	1669 (833)	1.5	0.0268

SEM: standard error of the mean.

[a] Relative fluorescent unit.

Table 1. Levels of cytokines in stage I/II versus stage III/IV ovarian cancer ascites.

Therefore, disrupting specific factors in cell-free ascites may provide an additional level of therapeutic intervention.

5. How does the tumor environment affect EOC dissemination?

One of the reasons for unsuccessful EOC treatment is its insidious nature, resulting from an unusual mechanism of dissemination. In contrast to other tumors that spread predominantly through lymph and bloodstream, EOC has a distinct tendency for metastasizing via shedding of cancer cells from the primary tumor site into the peritoneal cavity and implanting onto the mesothelial lining of the peritoneal cavity. The current admitted model for pelvic and peritoneal metastasis involves the shedding of tumor cells from the primary tumor into the abdominal cavity, wherein they survive and travel as free-floating multicellular spheroids to disseminate at distant sites where they adhere onto the mesothelial lining of the peritoneum and disaggregate to form metastatic outgrowth (**Figure 2**). Although not clearly define, each of these steps must require adaptive changes in tumor and/or stromal cells to progress to the next step.

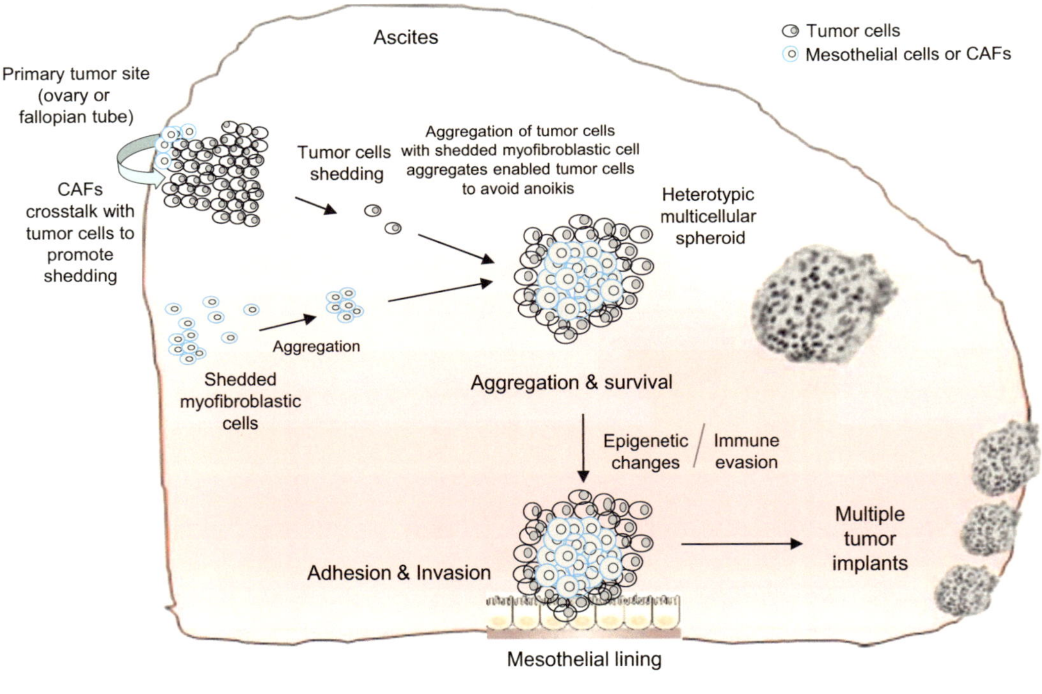

Figure 2. Model for EOC dissemination. CAFs in the primary tumor become educated by the tumor cells to acquire pro-tumorigenic functions. CAFs then in turns secrete a plethora of factors that enable tumor cells to exfoliate from the primary tumor. Once in the peritoneal fluid, tumor cells aggregate with free-floating mesothelial cells to form multicellular heterotypic spheroids, which enables tumor cells to avoid anoikis and gain a more invasive phenotype. Multicellular spheroids then attach to the mesothelial lining using various cell adhesion molecules. Mesothelial cells lining the peritoneum dissociate which enables tumor cells to invade to mesothelium lining.

A single mesothelial cell layer lines the pelvic and peritoneal organs including the diaphragm, bowel serosa, omentum and entire peritoneum. This mesothelial layer is highly receptive to ovarian cancer seeding [66]. Implantation of spheroids on the peritoneum involves interactions between cancer cells and the mesothelium. Adhesion of ovarian cancer cells to the mesothelial layer is facilitated by the expression of matrix metalloproteinase such as MMP-2 and MMP-9, and by fibronectin and vitronectin as well as their integrin receptors [67–69]. Once tumor cells have attached to the peritoneal surface, they gain access to the submesothelial environment by exerting force on the mesothelial lining, driving migration and clearance of the mesothelial cells [70]. Tumor cells undergo epithelial-to-mesenchymal transition (EMT) during the process [71].

Cells shed from the primary tumor aggregate to form free-floating multicellular spheroids in ascites, which initially spread to adjacent organs such as uterus, contralateral adnexa, bladder and rectum (stage II). After extension to the pelvic cavity, EOC will disseminate throughout a transcoelonic route to the peritoneal cavity forming multiple tumor implants (stage III), which are often difficult to remove completely at the time of the cytoreductive surgery and, substantially contribute to the high morbidity associated with this cancer. Metastasis can also occur beyond the abdominal cavity (stage IV). Whether the metastatic characteristics are already inherent in the primary tumor or are present only in subclone of metastatic cells within the primary tumor mass or occur in response to environmental cues remains unclear. This process of transcolonic seeding could be a continuing metastatic adaptive behavior or a passive process, in which exfoliated tumor cells that have already acquired all the necessary metastatic characteristics are merely transported via ascites into the peritoneal cavity to new sites. Comparative genomic studies showed similar genetic alterations in primary ovarian tumors and their respective metastasis supporting a passive transcolonic dissemination. However, transcriptomic analysis of matched primary tumors and peritoneal metastasis demonstrated the upregulation of certain pathways in metastatic lesions which suggest that the heterogeneity of tumor cells found in EOC is imposed, at least in part, by the nature of their surrounding environment [72]. The same group identified versican as a key upregulated gene in CAFs associated with the primary tumor, which promoted the motility and invasion of EOC cells by activating the nuclear factor-κB (NF-κB) signaling pathway and upregulating CD44, MMP-9, and hyaluronan-mediated motility receptor expression in cancer cells [73]. Versican expression was modulated by the activation of TGF-β signaling in CAFs induced by TGF-β ligands secreted by cancer cells. Therefore, these data further support the idea that ascites play an active, rather than a passive, role in EOC dissemination.

6. What are the effects of ascites on tumor cells?

The observation that ascites is often associated with the most invasive malignant tumors indirectly supports the notion that ascites is involved in the progression of EOC. Although different soluble factors in ascites have been implicated in EOC cell migration and invasion, the combined effect of the various factors found in cell-free ascites is also important to assess. Puiffe and colleagues have assessed the effect of 54 distinct ascites on growth, invasion and spheroid formation in comparison to serum in a single cell line [23]. They showed that ascites fell into one of two categories: stimulatory or inhibitory. The mechanisms or factors responsible for these opposite effects were not further investigated. Consistent with the results of Puiffe et al., Lane et al. showed that not all EOC ascites tested (2/6) promoted cancer cell migration [29]. In this study, the authors found that CCL18 was one of the factors in ascites implicated in ascites-induced cell migration. As such, CCL18 might represent a potentially new target in EOC treatment.

HGSOC ascites possess pro-survival properties. Ascites inhibits drug and TRAIL-induced apoptosis in EOC cells. Unsurprisingly, given the heterogeneity of ascites, the magnitude of the effects varies depending on the cell line and ascites tested [74, 75]. Multiple signaling pathways are activated by ascites in cancer cells, including up-regulation of anti-apoptotic protein Mcl-1 through ERK1/2-Elk-1 [76], up-regulation of anti-apoptotic protein c-FLIP [74], and activation of Akt through αvβ5/FAK signaling [75, 77], all of which contributing to the pro-survival effect of ascites. Collectively, these data support the notion that ascites is a tumor environment enriched with pro-tumorigenic molecules. A considerable effort is required however to gain a comprehensive understanding of how the different factors in ascites may alter the properties of tumor and stromal cells. The complexity of these processes requires the development of models that reflect the *in vivo* conditions as close as possible.

7. How can we exploit ascites for developing new therapeutic strategies?

More effective therapies to combat metastatic disease are urgently required for EOC, particularly in the context where early detection of this disease remain a difficult goal to achieve. Since the prognosis of patients with peritoneal metastases is directly correlated with optimal surgical cytoreduction [78], and widespread metastases are not often entirely amenable to surgery, the development of novel strategies to limit or stop metastatic progression is imperative. In that context, novel strategies that target interactions between cancer cells and their environment and inflammation-driven modifications are likely to be broadly applicable to cancers that metastasize within the abdominal cavity. In addition, as stromal cells are genetically more stable compared to tumor cells, targeting stromal cells rather than tumor cells would be less prone to the development of resistance. Thus, targeting the tumor environment may be a more compelling option.

Based on our increasing knowledge of the role of ascites and its components, a number of targeted specific therapies have been developed to improve EOC outcome. Bevacizumab, an anti-VEGF targeted therapy, is probably the most studied VEGF-targeting agent in EOC patients in the setting of front-line, maintenance or salvage therapy [79]. Although VEGF-targeting agents have yielded promising results in EOC in the settings of front-line and salvage treatment, the efficacy of these agents has yet to be clarified. Therapies taking advantage of the immune system could represent another potential avenue. For example, intra-peritoneal infusion of Catumaxomab, an anti-epithelial cell adhesion molecule (EpCAM), provided a significant improvement of ascites-related signs and symptoms [80]. Catumaxomab mediates a T-cell-induced lysis of tumor cells. Abagovomab is a murine monoclonal anti-idiotypic antibody that mimics parts of CA125. It is designed to act as an active immunogen aimed at breaking immune tolerance to the antigen. Unfortunately, abagovomab showed no improvement in progression-free or overall survival in a phase III clinical trial [81]. Another anti-CA125 antibody, Oregovomab, also failed to show improved outcome in EOC patients [82]. Anti-IL6 chimeric antibody Siltuximab has been assessed in phase II clinical trial but has shown very limited clinical benefits [83]. Other emerging strategies include the concept of neutralizing tumor-associated chronic inflammation as ascites in a highly pro-inflammatory environment [84].

8. Conclusions and future directions

There is an increasing interest for understanding the role of the tumor environment in the context of ovarian cancer. Recent studies have revealed new biological concepts and identified new therapeutic strategies to target the ascites. As illustrated by the limited clinical success obtained thus far, many challenges remain, including how to identify and target susceptible molecules given the complexity and heterogeneity of the tumor environment. Although the heterogeneity of ascites is a potential limitation, it also provides a unique opportunity for the development of personalized medicine based on the patient's characteristics. In that context, the profiling of the cell-free ascites components could guide clinical decision making for patient management. An important aspect to overcome limitations to unsuccessful clinical trials is the development and implementation of suitable *in vitro* and *in vivo* pre-clinical models that accurately mirror the clinical situation. For example, mounting evidence suggests that cell behavior in 3D cultures differs from monolayer cultures and better reflects the *in vivo* situation.

The accessibility of ascites translates into a readily available source of proximal fluids. In that context, ascites is a milieu from which we could potentially derive diagnostic and prognostic biomarkers. With the advances in our understanding of the crosstalk between the different cellular components of ascites and the various cues that cells receive from the surrounding environment, it is anticipated that reliable biomarkers will become available in the near future.

Acknowledgements

This work was supported by internal funding from Université de Sherbrooke.

Conflict of interest statement

Author declares no conflict of interests for this article.

Author contribution

Piché A. drafted the paper and wrote the final version. Matte I. and Bessette P. reviewed the draft and approved the final version.

Author details

Isabelle Matte[1], Paul Bessette[2] and Alain Piché[1]*

*Address all correspondence to: alain.piche@usherbrooke.ca

1 Département de Microbiologie et Infectiologie, Faculté de Médecine, Université de Sherbrooke, Sherbrooke, Canada

2 Département de Chirurgie, Faculté de Médecine, Université de Sherbrooke, Sherbrooke, Canada

References

[1] Siegel RL, Miller KD, Jemal A. Cancer Statistics 2017. CA: A Cancer Journal for Clinicians. 2017;**67**:7-30. DOI: 10.3322/caac.21387

[2] Ozols RF, Bookman MA, Connolly DC, Daly MB, Godwin AK, Schilder RJ, Xu X, Hamilton TC. Focus on epithelial ovarian cancer. Cancer Cell. 2004;**5**:19-24. DOI: 10.1016/S1535-6108(04)00002-9

[3] Bast RC, Hennessy B, Mills GB. The biology of ovarian cancer: New opportunities for translation. Nature Reviews. Cancer. 2009;**9**:415-428. DOI: 10.1038/nrc2644

[4] Shen-Gunther J, Mannel RS. Ascites as a predictor of ovarian malignancy. Gynecologic Oncology. 2002;**87**:77-83. DOI: 10.1006/gyno.2002.6800

[5] Ayhan A, Gultekin M, Taskiran C, Dursun P, Firat P, Bozdag G, Celik NY, Yuce K. Ascites and epithelial ovarian cancers: A reappraisal with respect to different aspects. International Journal of Gynecological Cancer. 2007;**17**:68-75. DOI: 10.1111/j.1525-1438.2006.00777.x

[6] Kobel M, Kalloger SE, Boyd N, McKinney S, Mehl E, Palmer C, Leung S, Bowen NJ, Ionescu DN, Rajput A, Prentice LM, Miller D, Santos J, Swenerton K, Gilks CB, Huntsman D. Ovarian carcinoma subtypes are different diseases: Implications for biomarker studies. PLoS Medicine. 2008;**5**:e232. DOI: 10.1371/journal.pmed.0050232

[7] Ramalingam P. Morphologic, immunophenotypic, and molecular features of epithelial ovarian cancer. Oncology (Williston Park). 2016;**30**:166-176

[8] Tan DS, Agarwal R, Kaye SB. Mechanisms of transcoelomic metastasis in ovarian cancer. Lancet Oncol. 2006;**7**:925-934. DOI: 10.1016/S1470-2045(06)70939-1

[9] Poveda VA, Casado HA, Cervantes RA, Gallardo RD, Garcia GE, Gonzalez MA, Lopez GG, Mendiola FC, Ojeda GB. Treatment guidelines in ovarian cancer. Clinical & Translational Oncology. 2007;**9**:308-316. DOI: 10.1007/s12094-007-0058-8

[10] Hanahan D, Coussens LM. Accessories to the crime: Functions of cells recruited to the tumor microenvironment. Cancer Cell. 2012;**21**:309-322. DOI: 10.1016/j.ccr.2012.02.022

[11] Swartz MA, Lida N, Roberts EW, Sangaletti S, Wong MH, Yull FE, Coussens LM, DeClerck YA. Tumor microenvironment complexity: Emerging roles in cancer therapy. Cancer Research. 2012;**72**:2473-2480. DOI: 10.1158/0008-5472.CAN-12-0122

[12] Quail DF, Joyce JA. Microenvironmental regulation of tumor progression and metastasis. Nature Medicine. 2013;**19**:1423-1437. DOI: 10.1038/nm.3394

[13] Senger DR, Galli SJ, Dvorak AM, Perruzzi CA, Harvey VS, Dvorak HF. Tumor cells secrete a vascular permeability factor that promotes accumulation of ascites fluids. Science. 1983;**219**: 983-985. DOI: 10.1126/science.6823562

[14] Olson TA, Mohanraj D, Carson LF, Ramakrishnan S. Vascular permeability factor gene expression in normal and neoplastic human ovaries. Cancer Research. 1994;**54**:276-280 DOI: Published January 1994

[15] Kipps E, Tan DS, Kaye SB. Meeting the challenge of ascites in ovarian cancer: New avenues for therapy and research. Nature Reviews. Cancer. 2013;**13**:273-282. DOI: 10.1038/nrc3432

[16] Erez N, Truitt M, Olson P, Arron ST, Hanahan D. Cancer-associated fibroblasts are activated in incipient neoplasia to orchestrate tumor-promoting inflammation in an NF-kB-dependent manner. Cancer Cell. 2010;**17**:135-147. DOI: 10.1016/j.ccr.2009.12.041

[17] Ren J, Xiao YJ, Singh LS, Zhao X, Zhao Z, Feng L, Rose TM, Prestwich GD, Xu Y. Lysophosphatidic acid is constitutively produced by human peritoneal mesothelial cells and enhances adhesion, migration, and invasion of ovarian cancer cells. Cancer Research. 2006;**66**:3006-3014. DOI: 10.1158/0008-5472.CAN-05-1292

[18] Pasquet M, Glozio M, Mery E, Rafii A, Benabbou N, Mirshahi P, Hennebelle I, Bourin P, Allal B, Teissie J, Mirshahi M, Couderc B. Hospicells (ascites-derived stromal cells) promote tumorigenecity and angiogenesis. International Journal of Cancer. 2010;**126**:2090-2101. DOI: 10.1002/ijc.24886

[19] Matte I, Lane D, Bachvarov D, Rancourt C, Piché A. Role of malignant ascites on human mesothelial cells and their gene expression profiles. BMC Cancer. 2014;**14**:288. DOI: 10.1186/1471-2407-14-288

[20] Mills GB, May C, Hill M, Campbell S, Shaw P, Marks A. Ascitic fluid from human ovarian cancer patients contains growth factors necessary for intraperitoneal growth of human ovarian adenocarcinoma cells. The Journal of Clinical Investigation. 1990;**86**:851-855. DOI: 10.1172/JCI114784

[21] Richardson M, Gunawan J, Hatton MW, Seidlitz E, Hirte HW, Singh G. Malignant ascites fluids (MAF), including ovarian cancer-associated MAF, contains angiostatin and other factor(s) which inhibit angiogenesis. Gynecologic Oncology. 2002;**86**:279-287. DOI: 10.1006/gyno.2002.6760

[22] Yamada T, Sato K, Komachi M, Malchinkhuu E, Tobo M, Kimura T, Kuwabara A, Yanagita Y, Ikeya T, Tanahashi Y, Ogawa T, Ohwada S, Morishita Y, Ohta H, Im DS,

Tamoto K, Tomura H, Okajima F. Lysophosphatidic acid (LPA) in malignant ascites stimulates motility of human pancreatic cancer cells through LPA1. The Journal of Biological Chemistry. 2004;**279**:6595-6605. DOI: 10.1074/jbc.M308133200

[23] Puiffe ML, Le Page C, Filali-Mouhim A, Zietarska M, Ouellet V, Tonin PN, Chevrette M, Provencher DM, Mes-Masson AM. Characterization of ovarian cancer ascites on cell invasion, proliferation, spheroid formation, and gene expression in an in vitro model of epithelial ovarian cancer. Neoplasia. 2007;**9**:820-829. DOI: 10.1593/neo.07472

[24] Giuntoli RL, Webb TJ, Zoso A, Rogers O, Diaz-Montes TP, Bristow RE, Oelke M. Ovarian cancer-associated ascites demonstrates altered immune environment: Implications for antitumor immunity. Anticancer Research. 2009;**29**:2875-2884

[25] Matte I, Lane D, Laplante C, Rancourt C, Piché A. Profiling of cytokines in human epithelial ovarian cancer ascites. American Journal of Cancer Research. 2012;**2**:566-580

[26] Byrne AT, Ross L, Holash J, Nakanishi M, Hu L, Hofmann JI, Yancopoulos GD, Jaffe RB. Vascular endothelial growth factor-trap decreases tumor burden, inhibits ascites, and causes dramatic vascular remodeling in an ovarian model. Clinical Cancer Research. 2003;**9**:5721-5728

[27] Nakamura M, Ono YJ, Kanemura M, Tanaka T, Hayashi M, Terai Y, Ohmichi M. Hepatocyte growth factor secreted by ovarian cancer cells stimulates peritoneal implantation via the mesothelial-mesenchymal transition of the peritoneum. Gynecologic Oncology. 2015;**139**:345-354. DOI: 10.1016/j.ygyno.2015.08.010

[28] Matte I, Lane D, Laplante C, Garde-Granger P, Rancourt C, Piché A. Ovarian cancer ascites enhance the migration of patient-derived peritoneal mesothelial cells via cMet pathway through HGF-dependent and –independent mechanisms. International Journal of Cancer. 2015;**137**:289-298. DOI: 10.1002/ijc.29385

[29] Lane D, Matte I, Laplante C, Garde-Granger P, Carignan A, Bessette P, Rancourt C, Piché A. CCL18 from ascites promotes ovarian cancer cell migration through proline-rich tyrosine kinase 2 signaling. Molecular Cancer. 2016;**15**:58. DOI: 10.1186/s12943-016-0542-2

[30] Kassis J, Klominek J, Kohn EC. Tumor microenvironment: What can effusions teach us? Diagnostic Cytopathology. 2005;**33**:316-319. DOI: 10.1002/dc.20280

[31] Yung S, Chan TM. Pathophysiology of the peritoneal membrane during peritoneal dialysis: The role of hyaluronan. Journal of Biomedicine & Biotechnology. 2011;**180**:594. DOI: 10.1155/2011/180594

[32] Lopez-Cabrera M. Mesenchymal conversion of mesothelial cells is a key event in the pathophysiology of the peritoneum during peritoneal dialysis. Advances in Medical Sciences. 2014;**473**:134. DOI: 10.1155/2014/473134

[33] Rynne-Vidal A, Jimenez-Heffernan JA, Fernandez-Chacon C, Lopez-Cabrera M, Sandoval P. The mesothelial origin of carcinoma associated-fibroblasts in peritoneal metastasis. Cancer. 2015;**7**:1994-2011. DOI: 10.3390/cancers7040872

[34] Loureiro J, Aguilera A, Selgas R, Sandoval P, Albar-Vizcaino P, Perez-Lozano ML, Ruiz-Carpio V, Majano PL, Lamas S, Rodriguez-Pascual F, Borras-Cuesta F, Dotor J, Lopez-Cabrera M. Blocking TGF-β1 protects the peritoneal membrane form dialysate-induced damage. Journal of the American Society of Nephrology. 2011;**22**:1682-1695. DOI: 10.1681/ASN.2010111197

[35] Kajiyama H, Kikkawa F, Maeda O, Suzuki T, Ino K, Mizutani S. Increased expression of dipeptidyl peptidase IV in human mesothelial cells by malignant ascites from ovarian carcinoma patients. Oncology. 2002;**63**:158-165. DOI: 10.1159/000063801

[36] Havre PA, Abe M, Urasaki Y, Ohnuma K, Morimoto C, Dang NH. The role of CD36/dipeptidyl peptidase IV in cancer. Frontiers in Bioscience. 2008;**13**:1634-1645

[37] Stadlmann S, Amberger A, Polheimer J, Gastl G, Offner FA, Margreiter R, Zeimet AG. Ovarian carcinoma cells and IL-1beta-activated human peritoneal mesothelial cells are possible source of vascular endothelial growth factor in inflammatory and malignant ascites. Gynecologic Oncology. 2005;**97**:784-789. DOI: 10.1016/j.ygyno.2005.02.017

[38] Matte I, Laplante C, Garde-Granger P, Bessette P, Rancourt C, Piché A. Ascites from ovarian cancer patients stimulate MUC16 mucin expression and secretion in human peritoneal mesothelial cells through an Akt-dependent mechanism. 2017; Manuscript submitted.

[39] Thériault C, Pinard M, Comamala M, Migneault M, Beaudin J, Matte I, Boivin M, Piché A, Rancourt C. MUC16 (CA125) regulates epithelial ovarian cancer cell growth, tumorigenesis and metastasis. Gynecologic Oncology. 2011;**121**:434-443. DOI: 10.1016/j.ygyno.2011.02.020

[40] Giannakouros P, Matte I, Rancourt C, Piché A. Transformation of NIH3T3 mouse fibroblast cells by MUC16 mucin (CA125) is driven by its cytoplasmic tail. International Journal of Oncology. 2015;**46**:91-98. DOI: 10.3892/ijo.2014.2707

[41] Rao TD, Tian H, Ma X, Yan X, Thapi S, Schultz N, Rosales N, Monette S, Wang A, Hyman DM, Levine DA, Solit D, Spriggs DR. Expression of the carboxy-terminal portion of MUC16/CA125 induces transformation and tumor invasion. PLoS One. 2015;**10**:e0126633. DOI: 10.1371/journal.pone.0126633

[42] Reinartz S, Failer S, Schuell T, Wagner U. CA125 (MUC16) gene silencing suppresses growth properties of ovarian and breast cancer cells. European Journal of Cancer. 2012;**48**:1558-1569. DOI: 10.1016/j.ejca.2011.07.004

[43] Giannakouros P, Comamala M, Matte I, Rancourt C, Piché A. MUC16 mucin (CA125) regulates the formation of multicellular aggregates by altering β-catenin signaling. American Journal of Cancer Research. 2014;**5**:219-230

[44] Latifi A, Luwor RB, Bilandzic M, Nazaretian S, Stenvers K, Pyman J, Zhu H, Thompson EW, Quinn MA, Findlay JK, Ahmed N. Isolation and characterization of tumor cells from the ascites of ovarian cancer patients: Molecular phenotype of chemoresistant ovarian tumors. PLoS One. 2012;**7**:e46858. DOI: 10.1371/journal.pone.0046858

[45] Casey RC, Burleson KM, Skubitz KM, Pambuccian SE, Oegema TR, Ruff LE, Skubitz AP. Beta 1-integrins regulate the formation and adhesion of ovarian carcinoma multicellular spheroids. The American Journal of Pathology. 2001;**159**:2071-2080

[46] Shield K, Ackland ML, Ahmed N, Rice GE. Multicellular spheroids in ovarian cancer metastases: Biology and pathology. Gynecologic Oncology. 2009;**113**:143-148. DOI: 10.1016/j.ygyno.2008.11.032

[47] Matte I, Legault CM, Garde-Granger P, Laplante C, Bessette P, Rancourt C, Piché A. Mesothelial cells interact with tumor cells for the formation of ovarian cancer multicellular spheroids in peritoneal effusions. Clinical & Experimental Metastasis. 2016;**33**:839-852. DOI: 10.1007/s10585-016-9821-y

[48] Condello S, Morgan CA, Nagdas S, Coa L, Turek J, Hurley TD, Matei D. β-Catenin-regulated ALDH1A1 is a target in ovarian cancer spheroids. Oncogene. 2015;**34**:2297-2308. DOI: 10.1038/onc.2014.178

[49] Sodek KL, Ringuette MJ, Brown TJ. Compact spheroid formation by ovarian cancer cells is associated with contractile behavior and an invasive phentoype. International Journal of Cancer. 2009;**124**:2060-2070

[50] Matte I, Laplante C, Garde-Granger P, Bessette P, Piché A. Ovarian cancer ascites promote tumor spheroid adhesion and invasion. 2017; manuscript submitted

[51] Yin M, Li X, Tan S, Zhou HJ, Ji W, Bellone S, Xu X, Zhang H, Santin AD, Lou G, Min W. Tumor-associated macrophages drive spheroid formatin during early transcoelomic metastasis of ovarian cancer. The Journal of Clinical Investigation. 2016;**126**:4157-4173. DOI: 10.1172/JCI87252

[52] Puls LE, Duniho T, Hunter JE, Kryscio R, Blackhurst D, Gallion H. The prognostic implication of ascites in advanced-stage ovarian cancer. Gynecologic Oncology. 1996;**61**:109-112. DOI: 10.1006/gyno.1996.0106

[53] Lane D, Matte I, Rancourt C, Piché A. Prognostic significance of IL-6 and IL-8 ascites levels in ovarian cancer patients. BMC Cancer. 2011;**11**:210. DOI: 10.1186/1471-2407-11-210

[54] Chen YL, Cheng WF, Chang MC, Lin HW, Huang CT, Chien CL, Chen CA. Inteferon-gamma in ascites could be a predictive biomarker of outcome in ovarian carcinoma. Gynecologic Oncology. 2013;**131**:63-68. DOI: 10.1016/j.ygyno.2013.07.105

[55] Lane D, Matte I, Garde-Granger P, Laplante C, Carignan A, Rancourt C, Piché A. Inflammation-regulating factors in ascites as predictive biomarkers of drug resistance and progression-free survival in serous epithelial ovarian cancers. BMC Cancer. 2015;**15**:492. DOI: 10.1186/s12885-015-1511-7

[56] Mikula-Pietrasik J, Uruski P, Szubert S, Moszynski R, Szpurek D, Sajdak S, Tykarski A, Ksiazek K. Biochemical composition of malignant ascites determines high aggressiveness of undifferentiated ovarian tumors. Molecular Oncology. 2016;**33**:94. DOI: 10.1007/s12032-016-0810-4

[57] Rifai N, Gillette MA, Carr SA. Protein biomarker discovery and validation: The long and uncertain path to clinical utility. Nature Biotechnology. 2006;**24**:971-983. DOI: 10.1038/nbt1235

[58] Hanash SM, Pitteri SJ, Faca VM. Mining the plasma proteome for cancer biomarkers. Nature. 2008;**452**:571-579. DOI: 10.1038/nature06916

[59] Kuk C, Kulasingam V, Gunawardana CG, Smith CR, Batruch I, Diamandis EP. Mining the ovarian cancer ascites proteome for potential ovarian cancer biomarkers. Molecular & Cellular Proteomics. 2008;**8**:661-669. DOI: 10.1074/mcp.M800313-MCP200

[60] Amon LM, Law W, Fitzgibbon MP, Gross JA, O'Briant K, Peterson A, Drescher C, Martin DB, McIntosh M. Integrative proteomic analysis of serum and peritoneal fluids helps identify proteins that are up-regulated in serum of women with ovarian cancer. PLoS One. 2010;**5**:e11137. DOI: 10.1371/journal.pone.0011137

[61] Bery A, Leung F, Smith CR, Diamandis EP, Kulasingam V. Deciphering the ovarian cancer ascites fluid peptidome. Clinical Proteomics. 2014;**11**:13. DOI: 10.1186/1559-0275-11-13

[62] Maccio A, Madeddu C. Inflammation and ovarian cancer. Cytokine. 2012;**58**:133-147. DOI: 10.1016/j.cyto.2012.01.015

[63] Lo CW, Chen MW, Hsiao M, Wang S, Chen CA, Hsiao SM, Chan JS, Lai TC, Rose-John S, Kuo ML, Wei LH. IL-6 trans-signaling in formation and progression of malignant ascites in ovarian cancer. Cancer Research. 2011;**71**:424-434. DOI: 10.1158/0008-5472.CAN-10-1496

[64] Chen XL, Nam JO, Jean C, Lawson C, Walsh CT, Goka E, Lim ST, Tomar A, Tancioni I, Uryu S, Guan JL, Acevedo LM, Weis SM, Cheresh DA, Schlaepfer DD. VEFG-induced vascular permeability is mediated by FAK. Developmental Cell. 2012;**22**:146-157. DOI: 10.1016/j.devcel.2011.11.002

[65] Shender VO, Pavlyukov MS, Ziganshin RH, Arapidi GP, Kovalchuk SI, Anikanov NA, Altukhov IA, Alexeev DG, Butenko IO, Shavarda AL, Khomyakova EB, Evtushenko E, Ashrafyan LA, Antonova IB, Kuznetcov IN, Gorbachev AY, Shakhparonov MI, Govorun VM. Proteome-metabolome profiling of ovarian cancer ascites reveals novel components involved in intercellular communication. Molecular & Cellular Proteomics. 2014;**13**:3558-3571. DOI: 10.1074/mcp.M114.041194

[66] Sodek KL, Murphy KJ, Brown TJ, Ringuette MJ. Cell-cell and cell-matrix dynamics in intraperitoneal cancer metastasis. Cancer and Metastasis Reviews. 2012;**31**:397-414. DOI: 10.1007/s10555-012-9351-2

[67] Moss NM, Barbolina MV, Liu Y, Sun L, Munshi HG, Stack MS. Ovarian cancer cell detachment and multicellular aggregate formation are regulated by membrane type 1 matrix metalloproteinase: A potential role in I.p. metastatic dissemination. Cancer Research. 2009;**69**:7121-7129. DOI: 10.1158/0008-5472.CAN-08-4151

[68] Kenny HA, Kaur S, Coussens LM, Lengyel E. The intital steps of ovarian cancer cell metastasis are mediated by MMP-2 cleavage of vitronectin and fibronectin. The Journal of Clinical Investigation. 2008;**118**:1367-1379. DOI: 10.1172/JCI33775

[69] Kenny HA, Chiang CY, White EA, Schryver EM, Habis M, Romero IL, Ladanyi A, Penicka CV, George J, Matlin K, Montag A, Wroblewski K, Yamada SD, Mazar AP, Bowtell D, Lengyel E. Mesothelial cells promote early ovarian cancer metastasis through fibronectin secretion. The Journal of Clinical Investigation. 2014;**124**:4614-4628. DOI: 10.1172/JCI74778

[70] Iwanicki MP, Davidowtiz RA, Ng MR, Besser A, Muranen T, Merritt M, Danuser G, Ince TA, Brugge JS. Ovarian cancer spheroids use myosing-generated force to clear the mesothelium. Cancer Discovery. 2011;**1**:144-157. DOI: 10.1158/2159-8274.CD-11-0010

[71] Davidowitz RA, Selfors LM, Iwanicki MP, Elias KM, Karst A, Piao H, Ince TA, Drage MG, Dering J, Konecny GE, Matulonis U, Mills GB, Slamon DJ, Drapkin R, Brugge JS. Mesenchymal gene program-expressing ovarian cancer spheroids exhibit enhanced mesothelial clearance. The Journal of Clinical Investigation. 2014;**124**:2611-2625. DOI: 10.1172/JCI69815

[72] Leung CS, Yeung TL, Yip KP, Pradeep S, Balasubramanian L, Liu J, Wong KK, Mangala LS, Armaiz-Pena GN, Lopez-Berestein G, Sood AK, Birrer MJ, Mok SC. Calcium-dependent FAK/CREB/TNNC1 signalling mediates the effect of stromal MFAP5 on ovarian cancer metastatic potential. Nature Communications. 2014;**5**:5092. DOI: 10.1038/ncomms6092

[73] Yeung TL, Leung CS, Wong KK, Samimi G, Thompson MS, Liu J, Zaid TM, Ghosh S, Birrer MJ, Mok SC. TGF-β modulates ovarian cancer invasion by upregulating CAF-derived versican in the tumor microenvironment. Cancer Research. 2013;**73**:5016-5028. DOI: 10.1158/0008-5472.CAN-13-0023

[74] Lane D, Robert V, Grondin R, Rancourt C, Piché A. Malignant ascites protect against TRAIL-induced apoptosis by activating the PI3K/Akt pathway in human ovarian cancer cells. International Journal of Cancer. 2007;**121**:1227-1237. DOI: 10.1002/ijc.22840

[75] Lane D, Goncharenko-Khaider N, Rancourt C, Piché A. Ovarian cancer ascites protects from TRAIL-induced cell death through αvβ5 integrin-mediated focal adhesion kinase and Akt activation. Oncogene. 2010;**29**:3519-3531. DOI: 10.1038/onc.2010.107

[76] Goncharenko-Khaider N, Matte I, Lane D, Rancourt C, Piché A. Ovarian cancer ascites increase Mcl-1 expression in tumor cells through ERK1/2-Elk-1 signaling to attenuate TRAIL-induced apoptosis. Molecular Cancer. 2012;**11**:84

[77] Lane D, Matte I, Laplante C, Garde-Granger P, Rancourt C, Piché A. Osteoprotegerin (OPG) activates integrin, focal adhesion kinase (FAK), and Akt signaling in ovarian cancer cells to attenuate TRAIL-induced apoptosis. Journal of Ovarian Research. 2013;**6**:32. DOI: 10.1186/1757-2215-6-82

[78] Deraco M, Baratti D, Laterza B, Balestra MR, Mingrone E, Macri A, Virzi S, Puccio F, Ravenda PS, Kusamura S. Advanced cytoreduction as surgical standard of care and hyperthermic intraperitoneal chemotherapy as promising treatment in epithelial ovarian cancer. European Journal of Surgical Oncology. 2011;**37**:4-9. DOI: 10.1016/j.ejso.2010.11.004

[79] Mabuchi S, Wakabayashi A, Kimura T. VEGF targeting agents in ovarian cancer. In: Farghaly SA, editor. Ovarian Cancer—Basic Science Perspective. Croatia: Intech; 2012. p. 335-354

[80] Heiss MM, Murawa P, Koralewski P, Kutarska E, Kolesnik OO, Ivanchenko VV, Dudnichenko AS, Aleknaviciene B, Razbadauskas A, Gore M, Ganea-Motan E, Ciuleanu T, Wimberger P, Schmittel A, Schmalfelt B, Burges A, Bokemeyer C, Lindhofer H, Lahr A, Parsons SL. The trifunctional antibody catumaxomab for the treatment of malignant ascites due to epithelial cancer: Results of a prospective randomized phase II/III trial. International Journal of Cancer. 2010;**127**:2209-2221. DOI: 10.1002/ijc.25423

[81] Sabbatini P, Harter P, Scambia G, Sehouli J, Meier W, Wimberger P, Baumann KH, Kurzeder C, Schmalfeldt B, Cibula D, et al. Abagovomab as maintenance therapy in patients with epithelial ovarian cancer: A phase III trial of the AGO OVAR, COGI, GINECO, and GEICO–the MIMOSA study. Journal of Clinical Oncology. 2013;**31**:1554-1561. DOI: 10.1200/JCO.2012.46.4057

[82] Berek J, Taylor P, McGuire W, Smith LM, Schultes B, Nicodemus CF. Oregovomab maintenance monoimmunotherapy does not improve outcomes in advanced ovarian cancer. Journal of Clinical Oncology. 2009;**27**:418-425. DOI: 10.1200/JCO.2008

[83] Angevin E, Tabernero J, Elez E, Cohen SJ, Bahleda R, van Laethem JL, Ottensmeier C, Lopez-Martin JA, Clive S, Joly F, et al. A phase I/II, multiple-dose, dose-escalation study of siltuximab, an anti-interleukin-6 monoclonal antibody, in patients with advanced solid tumors. Clinical Cancer Research 2014;**20**:2192-2204. DOI: 10.1158/1078-0432. CCR-13-2200

[84] Coussens LM, Zitvogel L, Palucka AK. Neutralizing tumor-promoting chronic inflammation: A magic bullet? Science. 2013;**339**:286-291. DOI: 10.1126/science.1232227